DEDICATION

This book is dedicated to the men and women facing the diagnosis of kidney cancer and their families. We hope that this review of kidney cancer will be helpful in making decisions about treatment and survivorship.

JOHNS HOPKINS
MEDICINE

Patients' Guide to

Kidney Cancer

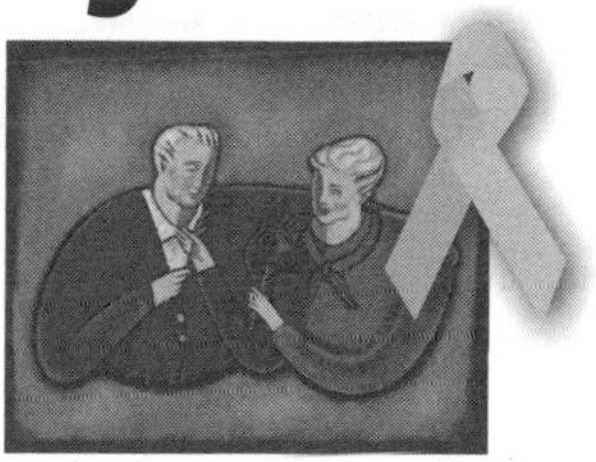

Janet R. Walczak, RN, MSN, CRNP

Nurse Practitioner in Urologic Oncology
Research Associate in Oncology
Sidney Kimmel Comprehensive Cancer Center at Johns Hopkins
The Johns Hopkins University School of Medicine

Michael A. Carducci, MD

Aegon Professor of Prostate Cancer Research
Professor of Oncology and Urology
Sidney Kimmel Comprehensive Cancer Center at Johns Hopkins
The Johns Hopkins University School of Medicine

SERIES EDITORS

Lillie D. Shockney, RN, BS, MAS

University Distinguished Service Assistant Professor of Breast Cancer; Administrative Director of Breast Cancer; Assistant Professor, Department of Surgery; Assistant Professor, Department of Obstetrics and Gynecology, Johns Hopkins School of Medicine; Assistant Professor, Johns Hopkins School of Nursing

Gary R. Shapiro, MD

Chairman, Department of Oncology
Johns Hopkins Bayview Medical Center
Director, Johns Hopkins Geriatric Oncology Program
The Sidney Kimmel Comprehensive Cancer Center at Johns Hopkins

JONES AND BARTLETT PUBLISHERS

Sudbury, Massachusetts

BOSTON TORONTO LONDON SINGAPORE

World Headquarters
Jones and Bartlett Publishers
40 Tall Pine Drive
Sudbury, MA 01776
978-443-5000
info@jbpub.com
www.jbpub.com

Jones and Bartlett Publishers
Canada
6339 Ormindale Way
Mississauga, Ontario L5V 1J2
Canada

Jones and Bartlett Publishers
International
Barb House, Barb Mews
London W6 7PA
United Kingdom

Jones and Bartlett's books and products are available through most bookstores and online booksellers. To contact Jones and Bartlett Publishers directly, call 800-832-0034, fax 978-443-8000, or visit our website www.jbpub.com.

Substantial discounts on bulk quantities of Jones and Bartlett's publications are available to corporations, professional associations, and other qualified organizations. For details and specific discount information, contact the special sales department at Jones and Bartlett via the above contact information or send an email to specialsales@jbpub.com.

The authors, editor, and publisher have made every effort to provide accurate information. However, they are not responsible for errors, omissions, or for any outcomes related to the use of the contents of this book and take no responsibility for the use of the products and procedures described. Treatments and side effects described in this book may not be applicable to all people; likewise, some people may require a dose or experience a side effect that is not described herein. Drugs and medical devices are discussed that may have limited availability controlled by the Food and Drug Administration (FDA) for use only in a research study or clinical trial. Research, clinical practice, and government regulations often change the accepted standard in this field. When consideration is being given to use of any drug in the clinical setting, the healthcare provider or reader is responsible for determining FDA status of the drug, reading the package insert, and reviewing prescribing information for the most up-to-date recommendations on dose, precautions, and contraindications, and determining the appropriate usage for the product. This is especially important in the case of drugs that are new or seldom used.

Production Credits
Executive Publisher: Christopher Davis
Editorial Assistant: Sara Cameron
Production Director: Amy Rose
Associate Production Editor: Jessica deMartin
Senior Marketing Manager: Barb Bartoszek
V.P., Manufacturing and Inventory Control: Therese Connell
Composition: Publishers' Design and Production Services, Inc.
Cover Design: Kristin E. Parker
Cover Image: © Image Club Graphics
Printing and Binding: Malloy, Inc.
Cover Printing: Malloy, Inc.

Library of Congress Cataloging-in-Publication Data

Walczak, Janet R.
  The Johns Hopkins patients' guide to kidney cancer / Janet R. Walczak and
Michael A. Carducci.
     p. cm.
  Includes bibliographical references and index.
  ISBN-13: 978-0-7637-7432-5
  ISBN-10: 0-7637-7432-4
  1. Kidneys—Cancer—Popular works.   I. Carducci, Michael.   II. Johns Hopkins
Medicine.   III. Title.   IV. Title: Patients' guide to kidney cancer.
  RC280.K5C38 2010
  616.99'461—dc22

                                                      2009022566

6048

Printed in the United States of America
13 12 11 10 09   10 9 8 7 6 5 4 3 2 1

Contents

Introduction: How to Use This Book to Your Benefit   vii

Chapter 1   First Steps—I've Been Diagnosed with Kidney Cancer   1

Chapter 2   My Team—Meeting Your Treatment Team   15

Chapter 3   Taking Action—Comprehensive Treatment Considerations   27

Chapter 4   Be Prepared—The Side Effects of Treatment   45

Chapter 5   Straight Talk—Communication with Family, Friends, and Coworkers   61

Chapter 6   Maintaining Balance—Work and Life During Treatment   67

Chapter 7   Surviving Kidney Cancer—Re-engaging in Mind and Body Health After Treatment   75

Chapter 8 Managing Risk—What if My Cancer   83
              Comes Back?

Chapter 9 My Cancer Isn't Curable—What Now?   87

Chapter 10 Kidney Cancer in Older Adults   93
              By Gary Shapiro, MD

Chapter 11 Trusted Resources—Finding Additional   107
              Information About Kidney Cancer and
              its Treatment

Information About Johns Hopkins   111

Further Reading   113

Glossary   115

Index   127

INTRODUCTION

HOW TO USE THIS BOOK TO YOUR BENEFIT

The goal of this book is to help you learn more about your cancer and make informed decisions about your care. By being better informed, we hope that you will be better prepared to confront the challenges ahead as you proceed through treatment and recovery. You will receive a lot of information from your healthcare team and will probably search the Internet or bookstores. No doubt friends and family members, meaning well, will attempt to give you advice about what to do and when to do it, and will try to steer you in certain directions.

Yes, your doctor has told you that you have kidney cancer. Although the diagnosis of kidney cancer is frightening, there is hope. There are more people surviving kidney cancer today than ever before. Hearing the diagnosis is difficult, but with support and accurate information to make good decisions, you can participate in the decision making about your care and treatment.

This book is designed to be a guide that takes you through the various treatment options and side effects and will help you put together a plan of action so that you become a kidney cancer survivor. The book contains information about current surgical and treatment options as well as recommendations for living with and surviving cancer. There is also a glossary in the back and resources listed for your further review and information. This information will help you to understand the how, when, and why of treatment options and make decisions with your doctors.

Let's begin now with understanding what has happened and what the first steps are to get you well again.

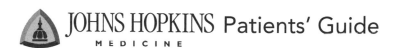

CHAPTER 1

JOHNS HOPKINS Patients' Guide
M E D I C I N E

FIRST STEPS—
I'VE BEEN DIAGNOSED WITH
KIDNEY CANCER

You have just been told that you have kidney cancer. You are shocked and can't believe that it can be true. Most people go through a wide range of emotions: disbelief, fear, loneliness, anger. This is normal. It's okay to have these feelings, to cry, and to be upset. But then, it's time to take action—to begin the process toward healing. Although you are the one with the disease, your family and friends will be affected too. But they can help you fight the disease.

Kidney cancer is a fairly common cancer with over 55,000 people estimated to be diagnosed each year. The number of new cases has risen each year over the past 5 to 7 years.

About one-third of those patients will have cancer that is confined to the kidney, another third will have locally advanced (involving a large part of the kidney and the surrounding area) cancer, and another third will have cancer that is metastatic, meaning that it has spread or traveled to other areas in the body. Of those patients who have their kidney removed due to cancer, about a third will develop metastatic kidney cancer from cancer that was not evident at the time of surgery. Although roughly 13,000 are expected to die each year from kidney cancer, it is estimated that there are over 200,000 kidney cancer survivors in the United States. It is expected that this number will grow as a result of people living longer with advanced kidney cancer. Most people with kidney cancer are between the ages of 40 and 70; there are almost twice as many men as women diagnosed. The most common type of kidney cancer is called clear-cell renal carcinoma and accounts for up to 70 percent of all kidney cancers. The second most common type is papillary renal-cell carcinoma and that occurs in about 10 to 15 percent of people. If kidney cancer is diagnosed early—before it has spread, chances of it coming back are low.

There are few symptoms caused by kidney cancer so it is usually not diagnosed until later when the tumor has grown large enough to press on other organs and cause symptoms that way. Some people are diagnosed when a tumor in the kidney is found when tests are being done for other reasons. The most common symptom of kidney cancer is blood in the urine. However, blood in the urine may be caused by other diseases such as kidney stones or kidney or bladder infections. So when blood is seen in the urine—especially in men, a doctor should be seen to determine the cause.

Other symptoms of kidney cancer include feeling a mass or hard lump or bulging in the abdomen, and pain or a feeling of pressure in the back or flank. However, back pain is a common symptom and doesn't usually cause concern until it is more continuous and increasing in intensity. There are other symptoms that can occur if the cancer has spread and depend on the areas involved. For instance, these may include weight loss that cannot be explained by diet or activity, fevers, anemia, high blood pressure, and increased calcium levels in the blood.

HOW TO SELECT YOUR ONCOLOGY TEAM AND CANCER CENTER

You want your team to be knowledgeable and experienced in the care of patients with kidney cancer. Don't rely on self-promoting advertisements on television as your way to select a facility and doctor. While you may seek out a comprehensive cancer center (look for one accredited by American College of Surgeons or National Cancer Institute), the important thing is that you select a facility that has kidney cancer specialists. These would include urologists that specialize in cancer surgeries (not general urologists or surgeons who rarely perform cancer-related surgery), medical oncologists who specialize in kidney cancer, radiation oncologists, urologic pathologists, radiologists, genetics counselors, oncology nurses, and psychosocial support staff for cancer patients. It's a highly specialized group. Your doctors and their staffs can be some of your best resources.

When you see your urologist, ask questions.

- How many kidney *cancer* surgeries do you do a year?
- What other types of surgeries do you do, and therefore how much time do you spend doing kidney cancer treatment?
- Are you board certified? In what specialty?
- How long have you been in practice?
- Do you regularly attend urologic cancer tumor boards to present cases for team discussion?
- Do you work with a multidisciplinary team of oncologists who also specialize in kidney cancer so continuity of care can be maintained?
- What is your philosophy on educating patients about their treatment options?

These are all questions you have the right to have answered before deciding that this doctor is to be your urologic oncology surgeon. If he or she hesitates answering them, consider that this person may not be the doctor you want to have performing your surgery.

It's not unusual for a patient to get a second opinion after an initial consultation, particularly if the initial consultation was at a facility where kidney cancer specialists may not be available or if there are still unanswered questions after the visit. Your doctor should not be offended by your seeking a second opinion. The second opinion may give you useful information and another perspective on treatment options. Your insurance company may in fact require that you seek a second opinion. If you need the name of a specialist, you can get names from the Kidney Cancer Association either by email request on their website (http://www.kidneycancer.org) or by calling them (1-800-850-9132).

LEARNING ABOUT YOUR DISEASE BEFORE THE FIRST VISIT

Let's start with some information about your cancer that will help you understand things better when you have your consultation. Initially, all information found on your medical reports and said to you will sound like a foreign language. However, by the end of your treatment, you will be quoting this information yourself with confidence and knowledge.

In kidney cancer, most people do not need to have a biopsy done because the kidney or part of the kidney will be removed. In some situations a biopsy may be performed to assist in the diagnosis. Most biopsies are fine-needle aspirates, meaning that a thin needle is inserted into the kidney mass and tissue is drawn up into the needle and syringe for pathologic review. This is usually done by an interventional radiologist who uses a CAT scan or ultrasound to guide the procedure. This piece of tissue gathered during the biopsy provides information about the diagnosis and type of cancer you have and a few specifics about its characteristics. It isn't intended to tell much more than this. All of the pathological information will be obtained at the time of the surgery.

The surgical removal of the kidney (nephrectomy) is the first treatment for most patients with kidney cancer who can tolerate the surgical procedure. Surgery is often recommended even if the cancer has spread at the time of diagnosis because there is some information that shows better survival if the kidney has been removed in the setting of metastatic disease. The nephrectomy will provide information about the type of kidney cancer and help to answer questions about prognosis, so it can be premature to ask the doctor too much about your prognosis, exact stage of disease (beyond what is called clinical staging, not pathology staging), and precisely what the details of your treatment will be until after your kidney has been removed. Putting together information from your kidney/abdominal imaging studies with or without the biopsy information provides what is needed to determine what your surgical treatment options will be.

After surgery, treatment or close follow-up will be determined by the pathology at the time of surgery and repeated scans. Side effects of the surgery and other therapies will be discussed in another chapter. Most patients after surgery return to their previous physical level and lifestyle.

GATHERING RECORDS: BIOPSY, RADIOLOGY STUDIES, OTHER TESTS

As soon as you are told that you have kidney cancer, request a copy of the scan report and pathology's biopsy summary report. Be sure to obtain copies of all of your medical records and request copies as you continue this journey so you can maintain your own portfolio of your care and treatment and test results. Begin with the initial scan or X-ray that found the mass on your kidney. If you have had a biopsy of the kidney mass or surgery, gather the pathology reports from both procedures. If you have had additional scans or X-rays, gather those reports and a CD of the scans as well. This could be an ultrasound, a CAT (computed axial tomography) scan, or an MRI (magnetic resonance imaging). No matter who sees you—urologic surgeon, medical oncologist, or radiation oncologist, they will want to review these. Although a report of the findings is helpful, it is also beneficial for them to review the actual films or images taken. Find out from the facility where the imaging was done how to go about picking up a CD and a report for the procedures and hand-carry them with you to your first consultation visit. Do the same with the pathology slides from your biopsy or surgery. You might think "why do I need to get these things if they have the reports," but an accredited cancer center is required to review the images and most specifically the pathology slides to verify their accuracy. There are situations in which a review by a urologic pathologist who specializes in this disease discovers that the pathology is different than was initially stated; meaning that it could change the recommendation for treatment. Accuracy is key for pathology. Your treatment plan at every step is based on this information being correct.

PATHOLOGY AND CANCER STAGING

Pathology and staging of cancers help your doctors better define your disease, prognosis, and how best to follow or treat you after the surgery. While some cancers are staged clinically, kidney cancer is mostly staged after the surgery is performed, when there is more information available from the pathologist about the primary kidney tumor and the extent of disease.

PATHOLOGIC DIAGNOSIS

As mentioned earlier, there are several types of kidney cancer. It is important to know exactly what type of kidney cancer you have because that will drive the choices for any additional treatment that you may need after your nephrectomy. Most kidney cancers are renal-cell carcinomas (90 percent) with the majority being the clear-cell type (70 percent). The next most common is the papillary type (10 to 15 percent). There are several other rare types such as the chromophobe, oncocytoma, collecting duct carcinoma, and unclassified renal-cell carcinoma (RCC). Another tumor involving the kidney is transitional cell carcinoma of the renal pelvis. This is not considered kidney cancer per se and is treated more like urinary bladder cancer. Each of these tissue types often have their own pattern of growth, spread, and progression that is associated with prognosis: Prognosis of the clear-cell type is related to the size or extent of the primary tumor in the kidney and how aggressive (the grade) the tumor is; similarly, the size and grade are important in prognosis of the papillary type. The papillary type that can be totally removed has an excellent prognosis but if it does come back, it is not as responsive to traditional kidney cancer treatments. The chromophobe and oncocytoma tissue types rarely metastasize or come back; collecting duct and unclassified types are rare but aggressive. There are also the medullary, sarcomatoid, and transitional cell types, all of which can be aggressive. The focus of this book is limited to the clear-cell and papillary types. However, if you have one of the other types of kidney cancer, most of the information may still be useful.

STAGING OF KIDNEY CANCER

The next piece of information determined by your medical team is the stage of your kidney cancer. Don't confuse stage with grade. This is a very common mistake, but they are quite different. Grade is related to cell growth and is a measure of the potential aggressiveness of the cancer. It will be discussed next. Stage determination combines several pieces of information (the size of the invasive portion of the tumor, nodal involvement, and other organ involvement) and is tied to survival estimates. Remember, however, that you are not a statistic; you are a person. A number of people need to fall on both sides of the statistics to produce these estimates, and you are embarking on doing whatever you need to do to be on the survival side.

Kidney cancer is staged from 1 to 4 and uses the TNM classification. The TNM classification looks at three components of the disease: T refers to the primary tumor, N refers to the lymph nodes, and M refers to metastasis. In order to determine the stage, these pieces of information are defined and then put together into a staging classification. First is the primary tumor in the kidney or the "T."

First is the "T," which refers to primary tumor in the kidney. It indicates the size of the tumor and whether it is confined to the kidney or has spread to surrounding tissues. The smaller the tumor, the lower the T number.

- Tx—Information not available about the primary tumor or cannot be assessed

- T0—No evidence of a primary tumor in the kidney

- T1a—Tumor less than or equal to 4 cm (less than about 2 inches) and confined to the kidney

- T1b—Tumor that is 4 to 7 cm (less than 3 inches) and confined to the kidney

- T2—Tumor greater than 7 cm but still confined to the kidney

- T3a—Tumor that has spread into the adrenal gland and into the tissue around the kidney

- T3b—Tumor that has spread into the large vein that takes blood from the kidney (renal vein) and part of the vena cava that takes blood up to and into the heart

- T3c—Tumor that involves the part of the vena cava up into the chest or actually is growing into the wall of the vena cava

- T4—Tumor that has spread through the Gerota's fascia (the tough wrapper around the kidney) and the tissue around the kidney

The next piece of information is about the lymph nodes or the "N" and tells you if none, one, or more of the lymph nodes close to the kidney are involved with the cancer. Sometimes, the lymph nodes are not surgically removed so that information may not always be available.

- Nx—Information not available or lymph nodes cannot be assessed

- No—No spread to the lymph nodes close to the kidney

- N1—Spread to one lymph node close to the kidney

- N2—Spread to more than one lymph node close to the kidney

Finally, the "M" tells you if there are any distant metastases present.

- Mx—Information not available or cannot be assessed

- Mo—No distant spread

- M1—Spread to other areas including distant lymph nodes or organs such as lungs, liver, bones, brain

All of this information is put together and summarized as stage 1, 2, 3, or 4.

Stage 1 cancer is confined to the kidney and is 7 cm (about 2¾ inches) or less. The cancer has not spread to other tissues, including the lymph nodes and other organs.

Stage 2 cancer is still confined to the kidney but is larger (greater than 7 cm or 2¾ inches) and, as in stage 1, has not spread to other tissues.

Stage 3 cancer is locally advanced. This means that the cancer could have spread to nearby lymph nodes, the adrenal gland (which is on top of the kidney), fatty tissue outside of the Gerota's fascia, or the veins but not to distant organs. In this stage, the primary tumor in the kidney can be of any size.

Stage 4 cancer is known as metastatic kidney cancer. Regardless of how large the primary kidney tumor is, the cancer has spread from the kidney and lymph nodes to other organs in the body, usually the bones, liver, lung, or brain. The presence of cancer in other organs is determined by scans and/or biopsies of these sites, where signs or symptoms were noted.

Other terms that you need to be aware of are clinical staging and pathological staging. Clinical staging is based on clinical examination findings and information gathered on scans, including measurements of the primary kidney tumor and the presence or absence of enlarged lymph nodes or the evidence of tumors or nodules of masses in other areas and organs. Pathological staging is more precise and is based on a pathologist actually measuring the diameter of the tumor once it has been removed at the time of surgery and looking under the microscope to see if cancer cells are in the lymph nodes and surrounding tissue.

GRADE OF KIDNEY CANCER

Once you know the stage and tissue type of the cancer, the next question is how aggressive is the tumor. This is the tumor grade. In kidney cancer, the cells are described using the Fuhrman system, which consists of grades 1 through 4 and is used to define how abnormal or unorganized the cells look under the microscope. Cells that are defined as grade 1 are those that look the least aggressive—closer to normal tissue—and tend to be slower growing and less likely to metastasize. At the other end of the spectrum is grade 4, which is more aggressive, faster growing, and likely to metastasize early. The higher the Fuhrman grade, the more aggressively the cells may act. Your pathology report will tell you the grade of your cancer. Don't be too taken with the grade though because it is just a number that doesn't really tell you how well YOU will do; it just helps your medical team to characterize your cancer and is simply part of the puzzle of putting together your treatment plan.

GENETICS OF KIDNEY CANCER

Although the vast majority of kidney cancers are not linked to any gene change or abnormality, about 5 percent of kidney cancers can be linked to gene changes. Most of the hereditary kidney cancers (about 75 percent) are of the clear-cell carcinoma type and are associated with a hereditary disease called von Hippel-Lindau disease or VHL. These kidney cancers usually involve both kidneys, are seen in younger people (under 40 years of age), and other family members have a history of kidney cancer. The gene involved in this disease has been identified (the VHL gene). People with VHL disease inherit the gene mutation but changes in this gene may also be seen in up to 60 percent of people with the sporadic type of kidney cancer. Normally, the VHL gene helps to suppress tumor growth through a variety of pathways that inhibit blood vessel growth (angiogenesis). However, when this gene can no longer function normally, it allows the pathways to in effect open and increase the production of growth factors that can lead to tumor growth. So the VHL gene can be a good gene but when there is a mutation or change in the makeup of the gene, it becomes a bad actor that allows tumors to grow. In fact, the biology of these genes has led to many of the treatment strategies doctors now use, specifically those targeting tumor blood vessel formation and growth-signaling pathways.

There are also two inherited forms of papillary kidney cancer. Hereditary papillary renal carcinoma (papillary type 1) involves the MET gene and accounts for about 5 percent of inherited kidney cancers. People with this type of inherited kidney cancer have an increased risk of multiple kidney tumors and an increased risk of developing tumors on both kidneys. Hereditary smooth-muscle tumors that are not cancerous (leiomyomas) and renal-cell cancer (papillary type 2) involve the FH (fumarate hydratase) gene and accounts for about 10 percent of inherited kidney cancer. This condition is associated with benign smooth-muscle tumors (leiomyomas) in the skin and, in females, the uterus, but also increases the risk of kidney cancer.

If it is suspected that you may have a hereditary type of kidney cancer, you should consider genetic counseling to determine if there is an increased risk of cancer for your children, or other family members. The counseling may help you to decide if and when you want to proceed with testing of you and your family members. In most cases of kidney cancer, there is no genetic risk identified. However, in those individuals/families where a risk is identified (the kidney cancer is in a person under 40, it involves both kidneys, and other family members have a history of kidney cancer or benign tumors), counselors will make a recommendation for you and your family members about screening measures and other possible preventative approaches if available.

CHAPTER 2

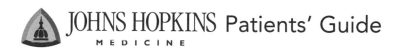

MY TEAM—MEETING YOUR TREATMENT TEAM

THE TEAM—UROLOGIC SURGICAL ONCOLOGIST, MEDICAL ONCOLOGIST, RADIATION ONCOLOGIST, RADIOLOGIST, PATHOLOGIST, NURSES, AND SOCIAL WORKER

Many people on your oncology team will be helping you to be well again. Each has a specific role and specialty related to kidney cancer and its treatment. The following is a list of the major players:

> *Urologic surgical oncologist.* A urologist is a surgeon who specializes in diagnosing, treating, and managing disorders of the urinary tract of men and women and the male reproductive tract. A urological surgical oncologist is a urologist

who specializes in cancers of the urinary tract, including kidney cancer, and performs the surgical removal of the kidney (nephrectomy). Some surgeons focus more on kidney cancer than others. This is usually the first doctor you will see if there is no question about the diagnosis or approach to treatment.

Medical oncologist. A cancer doctor who specializes in the medical treatment of cancers, including kidney cancer, and recommends medicines for systemic treatment that may include targeted therapy (treatment with the goal of blocking certain pathways or substances involved with tumor growth and development), immunotherapy, and chemotherapy. The consultation with this doctor is usually after you have recovered from your surgery, usually 2–4 weeks after surgery when the final pathology results are available. In many cases, if your risk for recurrence is low, you may not need a medical oncologist, but you can always ask for a referral and consultation. Occasionally, the medical oncologist is consulted if metastasis is suspected at the time of diagnosis. A joint discussion between the medical oncologist, urologist, and radiation oncologist may be necessary to define the optimal approach to treatment.

Radiation oncologist. A doctor who specializes in, treats, and provides recommendations for radiation treatments. This consultation is usually only needed for control of symptoms such as pain if the cancer has gone to the bone. Radiation is not routinely given in kidney cancer and has not been shown to be helpful after surgery to prevent the cancer from coming back.

Radiologist. The doctor who reads the scans, X-rays, and other images that are done to stage and follow your cancer.

Pathologist. Though you will probably never meet this person, he or she is one of the most important doctors on your team. He or she looks under the microscope at your biopsy tissue and your kidney cancer surgery tissue to determine the size of the tumor and whether the cancer has spread locally to the tissue surrounding the kidney or into the major veins, adrenal gland, and lymph nodes as well as providing important prognostic information that is used to determine your treatment plan.

Nurses. There will be several. You will probably meet new ones as you journey through your treatment, beginning with surgery, and followed by chemotherapy, radiation, and long-term care. Patient education, assessing your clinical needs, symptom control, administering anticancer drugs, and evaluating your progress during radiation if you need it are some of the functions they perform.

Social worker. This person helps arrange for any personal needs you may have, from assisting with financial issues, to arranging home health care (if necessary), to providing support networks.

MAKING YOUR INITIAL APPOINTMENT AT THE CANCER CENTER

The doctor you meet for your first consultation about your kidney cancer diagnosis will most likely be a urologist. But as discussed earlier, in some cases, if you have cancer that has spread, the first doctor with whom you meet may be a medical oncologist. The urologist should be a doctor who specializes in kidney cancer surgery. Many doctors call themselves urologic cancer surgeons but that doesn't mean they all are specialists or were trained as such. Knowing their credentials, board certification, volume of kidney cancer patients they treat, and asking them about some quality measures is useful information.

You want someone who does more than 25 to 50 kidney *cancer* surgeries a year. Note this didn't say "kidney surgeries." Biopsies are not to be included in these numbers, because often the urologist refers patients to an interventional radiologist to perform the fine-needle aspirate or biopsy of the kidney. You have the right to get these answers. If the doctor says he doesn't know how many surgeries he does, that may be a signal for you to seek guidance and treatment elsewhere. Most, if not all, physicians know the volume of kidney cancer patients they treat. It should not be a mystery.

Be sure that the person at the doctor's office helping to arrange your appointment knows that you are newly diagnosed with or suspected of having kidney cancer. They will do the best they can to get you a prompt appointment but they are also working with other patients like you who are newly diagnosed with cancer and wanting to be seen. Most facilities arrange for patient appointments quite promptly. It is not an emergency to be seen in the next day or two, although you may feel like it is; your kidney cancer has been there a little while. There are a few exceptions but only a few. This also means you have the time to make good decisions and be sure that you have yourself in capable hands. If the cancer center has a website, you might want to look at it and see if their faculty's background and specialty information are listed and if there is a particular doctor you think you may prefer to see over another.

Be sure to get clear directions and a specific address where you are to go and what time you are to report there. If you haven't been to this facility before, allow yourself extra drive time to find it, find parking, and get to the location where the doctor will be. Being late may frustrate you and may add to your anxiety. Arriving a little early gives you time to sit in the waiting area and review your questions one more time and take in deep breaths so your visit is as productive as possible.

You've got your appointment and directions where to go and what time to arrive. More than likely the scheduler you spoke with also provided you with instructions regarding what to bring. In case the information wasn't clear, the following is some information to help ensure that your visit is as productive and efficient as possible for you and the doctor you who will be seeing you.

WHAT TO BRING WITH YOU FOR THAT FIRST CONSULTATION

It's time for your first consultation with the urologist. Bring with you all those scans or X-rays that you have had done for the kidney mass/cancer; this includes CAT scans, ultra-sounds, and MRIs. The doctor may have requested that the pathology slides be sent by express delivery in advance with the goal that his or her pathologist would be able to look at them prior to your arrival and provide a diagnosis, which may vary from your original report. Also know in advance if your insurance company requires you to get preauthorization for having additional tests done, such as scans or ultra-sounds. There are situations in which the doctor reviewing the films finds them less than satisfactory or wants to have additional information. When this occurs, he or she may want to get additional imaging done either while you are there for this visit or at another scheduled time. Your surgeon may need to keep the scans and reports for a time and will use them during your surgical care. Most of the time, you will not need to worry about returning the scans because the CDs are duplicates and technically belong to you.

WHO TO BRING WITH YOU TO THE FIRST CONSULTATIVE VISIT

Bring a trusted family member or friend with you. When someone is stressed, they only hear and retain 10 percent of what is said to them. The doctor will be talking a great deal and you may feel overwhelmed trying to keep it all straight in your mind. The person with you serves as a scribe. You may bring a tape recorder with you as well. Most doctors are very comfortable with the discussion being voice recorded, but be sure you let the doctor know that you will be doing so before turning on the recorder.

WHAT ELSE TO BRING FOR THIS INITIAL VISIT

Be sure to bring an accurate list of what surgeries you have previously had and the details of any medical problems you have, such as prior kidney problems or infections, heart problems, lung problems, high blood pressure, thyroid problem, diabetes, and prior tumors (benign and cancer). You should also bring a list of the medications and the doses you are taking—prescription and over-the-counter (OTC) medicines including vitamins and herbs—as well as information about what allergies you might have. Also bring information about your family history for cancers, heart disease, diabetes, lung disease, and other serious illnesses. If you aren't sure, call another family member and recruit help in obtaining this information, because it is important for your medical summary and may provide information important in decision making about your treatment plan.

WHAT QUESTIONS TO ASK DURING YOUR VISIT

Having a list of questions prepared in advance is helpful in making the time you have with the doctor as efficient and optimal as possible. The following is a list to help you get started:

1. What type of kidney cancer do I have?

2. What stage of disease do you think I have based on what you know from my clinical examination, X-rays, and tests done thus far?

3. What type of surgery am I a candidate for? Total nephrectomy? Partial nephrectomy?

4. Did your pathology team confirm the biopsy results?

5. How many kidney cancer surgeries do you perform a year?

6. How long have you been doing kidney cancer surgeries?

7. How soon would my surgery be scheduled?

8. What educational information do you offer to prepare me for surgery and what to expect?

9. May I speak to a kidney cancer survivor volunteer who had the same surgery done here and had a similar treatment plan to what you plan for me?

10. Who will be my contact here for questions I may have? How will I contact that person?

11. Do you have educational materials for other family members, like my children?

12. Who else will be involved in my care and when will I meet them?

13. How soon after surgery will I see a medical oncologist?

14. Do you anticipate I will need additional treatment? If so, why?

15. Do you anticipate I will need radiation? If so, why?

16. How often will I be seeing you after my surgery for ongoing evaluation?

17. Are there any clinical trials that you would want to recommend for me to consider at this point?

18. Who will be coordinating my care? Do you have a patient navigator (someone dedicated to helping me through the system)?

19. How are subsequent appointments arranged for me and when do these happen?

WHAT TESTS NEED TO BE DONE: YOUR INITIAL WORKUP

As discussed earlier, not everyone will need a biopsy because most will undergo a partial or complete removal of the kidney. If you are able to have surgery, the diagnosis can be made at that time with the pathologic review and diagnosis of the tissue removed at the time of surgery. If you are unable to have surgery, a biopsy may be performed to confirm the diagnosis.

Because kidney cancer can spread locally and to other organs, you will need to have tests done to check your overall health and to see if any other areas are involved. The initial workup for the kidney mass would include a complete history and physical examination, blood tests to check your blood counts (complete blood count; CBC) to see if you are among other things anemic, chemistries (comprehensive metabolic panel and LDH) to check electrolytes and kidney and liver functions, and a urinalysis to further check kidney function. You will need to have a CAT scan of the abdomen and pelvis and a chest X-ray or chest CAT scan to define the extent of the disease in your kidney and to see if it has spread to other areas. The CAT scan is usually done with intravenous contrast and a barium solution that you drink that will better define the images of your organs. Another scan that might be performed is an MRI if the CAT scan shows that there could be a clot in the vena cava or low kidney function. It is also possible that you will have a bone scan if you are having persistent bone pain that isn't relieved with medicine and is increasing in intensity. A brain scan typically is not done unless you are having problems such as with balance or coordination, confusion or unclear thinking, or a persistent headache that could suggest that the cancer has spread to the brain.

HOW BEST TO CONTACT TEAM MEMBERS

Request business cards from each healthcare provider you see and ask what their office procedure is for responding to questions or concerns you may have. Usually there is one contact person you can rely on to serve this role. Also determine if you can communicate with any of the team by email. If and when the need arises that you have questions, be to the point and have your thoughts and questions written down when you call. It's better to ask three questions at once than one question three different times.

NAVIGATING APPOINTMENTS

Some cancer centers have patient navigators. The term navigator, however, is loosely defined and in some cases is used strictly for marketing and not really to navigate someone along their medical journey. When you inquire about this service, ask the process for assisting you with appointment scheduling, getting test results back, getting scheduled for your surgery, and seeing a medical oncologist after your surgery—in general being available for support and to address any other clinical needs that may arise. In some cases, your point person may be a nurse in the cancer center or an office manager in the doctor's office. In other instances, it may be a navigator or case manager. The title isn't important but the functions are.

FINANCIAL IMPLICATIONS OF TREATMENT/ INSURANCE CLEARANCE

You didn't plan on getting diagnosed with kidney cancer. No doubt this was not something that you ever thought you would be addressing for yourself. There is no convenient time to get this disease and the diagnosis alone can wreak havoc in your life. If you are working outside the home, you will be taking time off for your surgery and possibly for other treatment afterwards. Getting your ducks in a row early on is smart. Determining how much sick leave and short-term disability coverage you have and what your copayment information, prescription coverage, and other medical expense issues help in planning for your changing budget. Your insurance company may require referrals to be obtained in order to see certain specialists, get tests done, and get surgery authorized as well as other treatments or it may limit where these things can be done. If you need help with these things, ask for a social worker to assist you. In most cases, cancer centers also have financial assistants for this purpose.

There may be some treatments recommended that relate to clinical trials. Some may be covered by your insurance and others may not. If participating in a clinical trial, a research nurse will assist in getting this type of information answered for you.

If you lack health insurance, all is not lost. There may be resources available for people who need help and meet certain criteria for financial assistance and coverage of their cancer treatment expenses. Some states even have special grants for residents for precisely this purpose. Check with the social worker at the facility where you are being treated to get assistance and referrals. There are also organizations that provide transportation to and from treatment visits as well as food for you and your family, and even assist with the coverage of some medications. They aren't available in every state so rely on the social worker to tell you more about what is available for your geographic area.

Financial support services are not well advertised. It will require you to take the initiative to ask about them rather than waiting for someone to tell you about them. Be assertive and do this for yourself. That's why these programs exist. Money is the primary reason family members get into arguments. Avoid this upfront by discussing the issue and planning a budget. Be proactive in asking to meet with a social worker to discuss what support services are available for you as well.

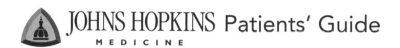

CHAPTER 3

JOHNS HOPKINS Patients' Guide

MEDICINE

TAKING ACTION— COMPREHENSIVE TREATMENT CONSIDERATIONS

This chapter will describe for you each of the various phases of treatment and the decision making involved in determining if you need that treatment. Kidney cancer treatment can include surgery, targeted therapy, immunotherapy, chemotherapy, and radiation therapy. The actual treatments that you will need depend on the type of kidney cancer, the results of surgery, and ongoing follow-up. Let's review each one now.

SURGICAL TREATMENT

Surgery remains the primary treatment for most kidney cancers and involves the removal of part of or the entire affected kidney. It has the highest cure rate (70–100 percent) in stage 1 and 2 cancer in which the cancer is localized to the kidney. The type of surgical procedure that you have depends on the type of kidney cancer, the size of the primary tumor, and if it has spread locally or to other organs. For most patients with kidney cancer, a total nephrectomy is done.

A nephrectomy is done when it is surgically possible; that is, when the tumor and surrounding tissue can be removed without serious risk. Patients who might not be candidates for total nephrectomy are those who have large, locally advanced cancer or metastases to multiple sites, have only one kidney, or have serious medical problems including heart, lung, liver, or other kidney disease. You should discuss the personal risks and potential benefits with your urologist or medical oncologist. They can help you to understand why surgery may be a good option for you. If you still have questions, or feel unsure about the options being recommended, get a second opinion.

There are two types of partial or total nephrectomy: the open approach, which is the more traditional approach, and the laparoscopic approach, which is often referred to as the "minimally invasive" surgery.

OPEN APPROACH

There are two types of open procedures, partial nephrectomy and radical nephrectomy. In the open partial nephrectomy procedure, through a surgical incision, the surgeon removes only the area in the kidney that is involved with the cancer. This procedure is used for a smaller primary tumor but also can be used if there is kidney failure, a problem with the functioning of the other kidney, or when someone only has one kidney. In the open radical nephrectomy, the entire kidney and surrounding tissue is removed via a large surgical incision. The radical nephrectomy is the procedure that is usually performed. It requires more extensive surgery and may include the removal of the adrenal gland that is just above the kidney as well as lymph nodes. The pathologist will look closely at all the tissue that is removed during surgery (the kidney, surrounding tissue, and, if removed, the adrenal gland and lymph nodes) to see if the cancer has spread microscopically. This can be quite extensive surgery, especially if the renal vein and vena cava are involved and require blood vessel (vascular) surgery. Vascular surgery, if needed, makes the surgical procedure longer, requires greater amounts of anesthesia, and involves more blood loss, often requiring transfusions. Your urologist will likely partner with a vascular surgeon if this is necessary. However, a nephrectomy is a fairly common procedure (with thousands performed each year for kidney cancer alone), and though there are certainly risks associated with the procedure—especially that of bleeding—overall deaths from surgery are only about 1 percent.

Even in advanced metastatic disease, the removal of the kidney is often indicated. There is some information that removing the kidney before having systemic treatment may be of benefit. This is particularly true when immunotherapy, such as Proleukin (interleukin 2, or IL2), and Intron A or Roferon A (interferon, or IFN), is the primary systemic treatment planned. It is not clear why this is true but it may be related to having less tumor volume for the body to have to fight. The primary kidney tumor does not always respond to systemic treatments and sometimes the metastases get smaller or go away after the kidney is removed. However, the downside of this is that the cancer may progress and get worse while you are recovering from surgery. Any complications could delay the time when additional treatment could be started for the cancer that remains. Thus, removing the kidney is usually indicated for patients who are good candidates for surgery: those who have a small volume of disease that has spread, but without spread to the brain or extensive spread to the liver or bone.

LAPAROSCOPIC APPROACH

A partial or radical nephrectomy can also be performed using the laparoscopic procedure. This procedure is a minimally invasive technique and involves inserting an instrument (laparoscope) into the abdominal cavity via small incisions to remove part of or the entire kidney. This procedure is used with increasing frequency because it is better tolerated by the patient, has a shorter recovery time, and the results are identical to the traditional open procedure. However, a radical nephrectomy via the laparoscope can be difficult to perform and may need to be converted to an open procedure to facilitate the nephrectomy and reduce the technical difficulty. This would involve making an incision so the surgeon can use a hand to help the laparoscope complete the procedure.

The partial laparoscopic nephrectomy has become a standard procedure for patients with renal-cell carcinoma who have small tumors (< 4 cm) that are located in the outer areas of the kidney, thus making them easily accessible. The results of a partial nephrectomy are less satisfactory in patients with larger renal-cell carcinomas, leaving the removal of the entire kidney as the standard approach.

ROBOTIC-ASSISTED SURGERY

Robotic-assisted surgery is a newer approach that has been employed in urologic surgery over the past few years. The potential advantage of the robotic-assisted procedure is the potential of improvement in the precision of the minimally invasive procedures such as the laparoscopic nephrectomy. The surgeon sits in a remote console and uses robotic arms and a laparoscope-type instrument to guide the procedure that uses small incisions into the abdomen. Advances in computer technology, digital equipment, and sophisticated robotic instrumentation have made this a viable option.

The advantages of the minimally invasive procedures over the open procedure are a decrease in blood loss and significantly less postoperative pain, a faster recovery with shorter hospital stays, a faster return to normal activities and work, and a more positive cosmetic result. Most medical centers offer this newer approach to the nephrectomy.

OTHER MINIMALLY INVASIVE APPROACHES

Cryoablation and Radiofrequency Ablation: Today, tumors are being discovered at smaller sizes and earlier stages. Removing small tumors without removing most of the kidney provides similar long-term cures as the complete kidney removal. Today's technology allows for the destruction of the tumors without having to physically remove them. Extremes in temperature, both heat and cold, can kill tumor cells. It is now possible to destroy tumors within the body by using X-ray guidance to place special needles or probes into the tumor that can deliver heat or cold energy inside the body. These needles freeze or heat the tissue to destroy tumors. This procedure is usually done by the staff in radiology and urology together to perform percutaneous tumor ablation without radical surgery. Cryoablation or cryosurgery involves freezing the tumor using liquid nitrogen or carbon dioxide to kill the cancer cells. Radiofrequency ablation uses heat to destroy the cancer cells.

Arterial Embolization: An arterial embolization is a procedure that involves the placement of a special sponge-like material into an artery that is supplying blood to the kidney involved with the cancer. This is done by inserting a thin tube catheter into a vessel in the leg and into the main vessel feeding the kidney. The sponge-like material is placed in the artery to block the blood supply that feeds the kidney and the tumor, hopefully causing the tumor to shrink. It can be used to potentially make the removal of the kidney and vascular surgery easier and control blood loss at the time of surgery, but it is more often used as a method of providing symptom control for someone who cannot undergo surgery. In this case, the pain or bleeding can be controlled with the arterial block or sponge-like material. Additionally, the sponge-like arterial block can by used to control the bleeding when metastatic disease to the bone is being operated on.

While all of these minimally invasive procedures are technically able to achieve the desired results, the long-term side effects and results are not known. Regardless of which type of surgical procedure is recommended, discuss the potential risks and benefits carefully with your surgeon.

Once the decision is made about what surgery treatment is best for you, you are likely to feel better knowing that you will now be taking action against the disease. No matter what surgical option is selected, you have taken your first step toward becoming a kidney cancer survivor!

RECOVERY

After surgery, you will need some recovery time. Deciding who will help you at home after surgery sounds simple but sometimes isn't. You may need some assistance at home with your daily activities, attending to wound care and such, and recovering from surgery and anesthesia in general. The length of time you need help will depend on the type of surgery you have. Ask the surgeon what to expect and request to meet with the nurse preoperatively to review teaching instructions so you are well prepared as to what to expect.

If other people will be coming to stay to help you, talk with them about roles and responsibilities before the surgery. Write out what each person is responsible for doing—buying the groceries, making dinner, tending to family responsibilities, and so on. Planning ahead prevents possible problems later on, but it is not foolproof. Function as a team—remember, this is a team effort! Remember, too, that the best-laid plans may need to be modified as the situation evolves and changes. You and the family member or friend who will be helping you need to talk about your expectations of each other.

You can expect to have some incisional discomfort that may require pain medication for a few days after discharge; after that, acetaminophen should be sufficient to control your pain. You could be told to stay on a no-added salt diet and avoid a high-protein diet because both can cause potential damage to your remaining kidney. While this is the usual recommendation, there are no data solid data to support it. Certainly, maintaining a diet that is well rounded and heart healthy with fruits and vegetables, low salt, and low animal fat can help to keep you healthy. Patients are encouraged to have an annual blood test to include a complete blood count, serum creatinine (to follow the function of the remaining kidney), and liver function tests performed by their primary care physician. Your surgeon will also review these results in the office during follow-up visits. Follow-up X-ray tests (e.g., CAT, MRI, sonograms) may be periodically required to follow the appearance of your remaining kidney.

It is best to discuss methods and guidelines to protect your remaining kidney with your primary care physician after fully recovering from surgery.

RESUMING PHYSICAL ACTIVITY AFTER SURGERY

You may shower after returning home from the hospital. Your wound sites can get wet, but must be padded dry immediately after showering. Tub baths are not recommended in the first 2 weeks following surgery because this will soak your incisions and increase the risk of infection. You will have adhesive strips across your incisions that will fall off in approximately 5 to 7 days on their own. The sutures underneath the skin will dissolve in 4 to 6 weeks. These are general rules. Talk to your urologist about your postoperative plan of care and activity.

Taking walks is advised; prolonged sitting or lying in bed should be avoided. Climbing the stairs is possible, but they should be taken slowly. Driving should be avoided for at least several weeks after surgery. Do not do any heavy lifting (greater than 20 pounds) or exercising (jogging, swimming, treadmill, biking) for 6 weeks or until instructed by your doctor. Most patients return to full activity at home on an average of 3 weeks following surgery. You can expect to return to work in approximately 4 weeks, but your urologist will give you the final okay and specific instructions for activities.

If you have an outpatient tumor ablation procedure that is done via the laparoscope, you should take it easy for the remainder of the day following the procedure. Most patients are able to resume full activities the day after the procedure. If you were on any blood-thinning medicine prior to the surgery, you should wait 48 hours before restarting the medication. If there is persistent blood in your urine, contact your physician prior to restarting these medicines.

SYSTEMIC TREATMENT

Systemic treatment (treatment that goes to all parts of the body) is usually given when the kidney cancer recurs or spreads to other areas of the body. It may be given orally (by mouth), intravenously (via a needle-like device into a vein), or by subcutaneous injection (injection under the skin) depending on the drug. There are several types of systemic treatment, including immunotherapy (Proleukin or Intron A/Roferon A), which are drugs that stimulate the immune systemic to generally fight disease or targeted therapy (Sutent [sunitinib], Nexavar [sorafenib], Torisel [temsirolimus], Afinitor [everolimus], or Avastin [bevacizumab]) that interferes with the action of specific molecule or cell growth pathways involved in tumor growth. Chemotherapy (Gemzar [gemcitabine], Xeloda [capecitabine], Adrucil [5-fluorouracil]) is a group of drugs that act on dividing cells to cause cell death and are not usually given in kidney cancer, but can be if other therapies fail.

Proleukin is usually only given to patients who have a good functional status and a small amount of metastatic clear-cell type cancer that is primarily metastatic to the lungs. It should not be considered if the patient has brain metastases. It is administered intravenously in high-dose regimens that require hospitalization, often in an intensive care unit. It nonspecifically activates the immune system to fight the kidney cancer. The side effects can be severe. They include extremely low blood pressure that can cause other problems if not treated aggressively with medicines to increase it. However, Proleukin can produce a complete response (where the cancer can no longer be seen on scans). This response can last for extended periods, but rarely produces a cure.

Intron A/Roferon A was once the primary treatment for renal-cell cancer but is now used less often. It is injected under the skin at home and is also nonspecific immuno-therapy.

Sutent and Nexavar are targeted agents and are considered first line therapy for most kidney cancers that are recurrent or have spread. These newer drugs are oral agents that work by blocking certain cell pathways involved in blood vessel growth; thus, they potentially inhibit blood supply to the areas involved with cancer. Sutent is most commonly prescribed for first-line therapy if the patient is not a candidate for immunotherapy. Nexavar may be used in some situations where patients cannot take Sutent because of decreased cardiac function. Torisel and Afinitor are also targeted agents, but they work by blocking pathways that are needed for production of key proteins required for tumor cell growth and survival and blood vessel growth. Torisel is given intravenously on a weekly basis while Afinitor is taken orally. These are typically used if the cancer is getting worse on Sutent or Nexavar. Avastin is a monoclonal antibody that targets growth factors involved in blood vessel growth. It may be considered in combination with Intron A/Roferon A as first line treatment or used later when the cancer is continuing to grow despite treatment. Avastin offers another treatment option for patients.

NEOADJUVANT SYSTEMIC THERAPY

Neoadjuvant systemic therapy is treatment that is given prior to surgery in an effort to reduce the amount of cancer that will need to be removed. It is not considered part of the standard of care for primary kidney cancer; however, there are special circumstances in which systemic therapy may be recommended as the first phase of treatment against kidney cancer. In any cancer, the goal of systemic therapy is to carry medicine to all parts of the body where the disease may be located, including, in this instance, the kidney and beyond to other sites of disease. This may be recommended for people with locally advanced disease requiring extensive surgery that is likely to be risky and to cause serious side effects. If the disease responds to the therapy and the tumor shrinks, the surgeon may then be able to remove the kidney and tumor with less morbidity. Although doctors have new drugs that can be given before surgery, this approach is not yet considered standard. Still, it is a trend to watch, and you may want to ask your doctor if it's an option for you.

ADJUVANT TREATMENT

For many cancers such as breast and colon cancer, "adjuvant treatment" after surgery is part of the standard of care. It is used when all known cancer has been removed, yet there remains a significant risk that the cancer will come back.

It is sort of an insurance policy to increase the chance that the cancer does not return or to delay the recurrence of the cancer. In kidney cancer, however, doctors have no data that systemic adjuvant therapy, such as chemotherapy or targeted agents, in this setting. Thus, in kidney cancer, adjuvant therapy still remains investigational, and most doctors will not recommend it as a standard. Currently, clinical trials are looking to see if newer targeted oral agents are useful for adjuvant therapy in kidney cancer. You may be asked to take part in a clinical trial depending on the results of your surgery: on the stage of the cancer, the type of surgery performed, the grade of the cancer cells, your general health, and other prognostic factors determined by the pathologist after examining the tumor itself.

TREATMENT FOLLOWING SURGERY

When you have recovered from the surgery, you will have scans done periodically over the next 5 years to see if you have any recurrent or metastatic disease. Some patients who develop metastatic disease can be followed with periodic scans to see if the cancer is slow growing. If it grows or spreads to new areas, your oncologist will discuss further treatment with you. If you had metastatic disease prior to surgery, the usual approach is to wait until you have recovered from the effects of the surgery before beginning any additional therapy. At that time, new scans will be obtained to assess if your cancer is growing. Only if your cancer is growing, and you are well, will your oncologist recommend additional treatment. (See **Chapter 8** for additional information.)

RADIATION

Radiation usually is not part of the initial treatment plan unless there is kidney cancer that has gone to (metastasized to) the bones. In that situation, radiation may be used with or without orthopedic surgery to treat pain and stabilize the bones. If orthopedic surgery is indicated, the area of cancer in the bone may require embolization similar to that discussed previously. Radiation doesn't hurt. It feels similar to getting an X-ray, which means you feel nothing at all. However radiation effects are cumulative; that's why you may start getting fatigued toward the last few weeks of treatment. Try to stay as active as possible during this time to help reduce this side effect.

CLINICAL TRIALS

New and innovative treatments are developed and implemented by doing clinical trials. Clinical trials help doctors to improve the treatment of kidney cancer by finding new agents or approaches to treating it; they are the backbone of science today. Your doctors may at any given time during your treatment discuss with you opportunities to participate in a clinical trial. Be open-minded. Hear what is being offered as part of a study. Let's begin by educating you about what is meant by the term "clinical trials."

There are many different types of clinical trials. They may range from studies focusing on ways to prevent, detect, diagnose, treat, and control kidney cancer to studies that address quality-of-life issues that affect the patient. Most clinical trials are carried out in phases. Each phase is designed to learn different information and build upon the information previously discovered. Patients may be eligible for studies in different phases, depending on their stage of disease and anticipated therapies, as well as treatment they have already had. Patients are monitored at specific intervals while participating in studies.

Phase I studies are the earliest phase of testing in people. These studies aim to discover the best way to do a new treatment, what the side effects are, and how much of the treatment (what dose and schedule) can be given safely; the study may or may not be kidney cancer specific. In such studies, only a small number of patients are asked to participate. They are often offered to patients whose cancer cannot be helped by other known treatment modalities or when existing therapies have limited activity and the patient and oncologist seek alternatives. Also, patients who have exhausted other treatment options may be candidates for a phase I trial. Some phase I studies may combine treatments that are already approved for kidney cancer but have not been given together before. (This type of phase I study is kidney cancer specific and may be offered to people much earlier in the disease.) Some patients have personally received benefit from participation, but others have experienced no benefit in fighting their cancer. They are, however, paving the way for the next generation, which is important.

Phase II studies are based on the dose and side-effect findings from the phase I stud and are designed to learn if the treatment works in patients with kidney cancer. (These studies

are typically cancer specific; in your case, the study would be focusing on kidney cancer.) The number of patients in this type of study is usually between 20 and 50. Patients whose kidney cancer no longer responds to other known treatments may be offered participation in this type of trial. These studies may also involve new agents being evaluated prior to standard or traditional therapies. Tumor shrinkage or clinical benefit (disease isn't growing or symptoms/pain are controlled) is measured and patients are closely observed to assess the effects the treatment is having on their disease. Phase II studies also closely monitor side effects and thus provide a record of side effects that occur.

Phase III studies usually compare new treatments (those that appear to be promising from phase II trials) with standard treatments or possibly a placebo. A placebo looks like the new study drug but does not contain any drug at all. The phase III study requires large numbers of participating patients, at least hundreds depending on the type of study, and is cancer specific (in your case, only for kidney cancer patients). Patients usually are randomly assigned to a treatment regimen group: to either the new approach or the standard one (or placebo). These studies seek benefits of longer survival, better quality of life, fewer side effects, and fewer cases of cancer recurrence. There are usually strict rules for being eligible for this type of study, such as type of kidney cancer (pathological type), prior therapy, and stage of disease.

Neoadjuvant and adjuvant studies are conducted to determine if additional therapy will further improve the chance for long-term survival and offer a reduction in the risk of recurrence. Neoadjuvant studies initially are used prior to surgical intervention and adjuvant studies are given after surgery. Because doctors currently have no data that either type of additional therapy is beneficial, these studies are important to test some of the newer agents. These studies are offered at the time of initial therapy and the main purpose is to prevent or delay recurrence. These studies progress through phases I, II, and III trials like other treatment studies.

Supportive care studies are tailored to improve ways of managing side effects caused by treatment. They include quality-of-life studies as well.

The following is a list of questions that you should consider asking that may help guide you in decision making and fact finding about clinical trials for the treatment of kidney cancer:

What is the purpose of the study?

What is the current standard of care?

How many people will be included in the study?

What does the study involve?

What kinds of tests and treatment will I have?

How are treatments given and what side effects might I expect?

Is there a placebo?

What are the risks and benefits of each protocol?

How long will the study last?

What type of long-term follow-up care is provided for those who participate?

Will I incur any costs? Will my insurance company pay for part of this?

When will the results be known?

Realize that an individual may derive substantial benefit from participating in clinical trials. Every successful cancer treatment being used today started as a clinical trial. Those patients who participated in these studies were the first to benefit. Participation can potentially benefit you, but perhaps equally important (and to some, more important), you may be contributing in a major way for subsequent patients having to deal with this disease.

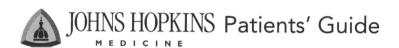

CHAPTER 4

JOHNS HOPKINS Patients' Guide

M E D I C I N E

BE PREPARED—THE SIDE EFFECTS OF TREATMENT

The side effects that a patient may experience while undergoing the primary treatment of their kidney cancer will vary depending on the type of treatment that is performed. Some side effects are easily controlled and some may be more difficult. No two patients are alike so don't assume if you knew someone with kidney cancer in the past that your situation will mirror image theirs. The following are some of the more common side effects that should be discussed with your oncology team so you have a head's up as to what to expect in relationship to the status of your disease and the treatment recommendations they are making on your behalf.

This list can look overwhelming. It is not intended to alarm you but rather to provide you with a thorough comprehensive list of possible issues that may need to be addressed while undergoing treatment. Although most will have surgery, not everyone will need systemic treatment, such as the targeted agents, or radiation. Whether needed now or in the future, you will have this overview to use as a reference when and if it is needed.

ANEMIA

Anemia is a common problem for many dealing with cancer and may be a side effect of the kidney cancer itself, the surgery (especially if an open procedure is done), or systemic therapy for advanced/metastatic disease such as immunotherapy and the targeted agents of Sutent, Nexavar, Torisel, Afinitor, and Avastin. By definition, anemia is an abnormally low level of red blood cells (RBCs). These cells contain hemoglobin (an iron protein) that provides oxygen to all parts of the body. If RBC levels are low, parts of the body may not be receiving all the oxygen it needs to work and function well. In general, people with anemia commonly report feeling tired. The fatigue that is associated with anemia can seriously affect the quality of life for some patients and make it difficult for patients to cope at times.

In cases of anemia related to the kidney cancer, the anemia will usually improve after surgery. When the anemia is a result of chemotherapy, anemia will usually improve after the therapy is stopped. Trying to eat a healthy diet may help. Your doctor may recommend taking an iron supplement. If the anemia is a result of chemotherapy, medications such as Procrit/Epogen (epoetin) or Aranesp (darbepoetin) may be recommended to stimulate your bone marrow to make more red blood cells, raising your blood cell count and increasing your energy level. Such a medication is given by injection under the skin using a very small, thin needle. Doses vary and it is common to be given one of these medications for this side effect once a week or every other week. Recently, there has been a great deal of controversy as to the benefits of these agents, so usage has dramatically declined. Talk to your doctor about whether this is indicated for you. You might be advised to also take an iron supplement orally while getting these injections.

FATIGUE

Feeling exhausted or extremely tired is probably the most common side effect patients report. This can happen as a side effect of the cancer, surgery and anesthesia, immunotherapy, systemic targeted therapy, and radiation therapy. Fatigue can also be triggered by anemia that can be treated to relieve or reduce this symptom. If there are specific problems you are experiencing that are related to fatigue (such as a difficulty in sleeping), make your doctor aware so that he might prescribe something to help you sleep better. Also ask about how to better cope with your emotional distress, which can increase fatigue.

Conserving your energy is important so you are able to spend your time doing things that are important to you. Make a list of the activities and chores you are trying to accomplish (food shopping, work, housecleaning, etc.) and spread your activities out through the day. See about recruiting help from family and friends to assist you with jobs such as housekeeping, laundry, yard care, and meal preparation so you can spend more time doing things you want to get done. You may also notice that your energy level is better during certain times of the day. You may discover that slowly increasing your activity levels (such as taking walks) will help to improve your endurance and energy level. Start out slow and gradually increase your distance and speed. Try to eat as healthy as you can, focusing on proteins and carbohydrates and maintaining an adequate fluid intake. If you get tired after an activity, sit down and rest or take a nap. The Oncology Nursing Society has a website that provides some specific recommendations related to this side effect. Take a look at http://www.cancersymptoms.org and click on fatigue.

HEART PROBLEMS

If you need to take systemic therapy, you will probably have at least one of the targeting drugs such as Sutent, Nexavar, Torisel, Afinitor, and Avastin. These drugs can have side effects that affect the function of the heart. This can cause congestive heart failure, a weakness of the heart muscle, but is not common. The key is close monitoring, and for you to report any symptoms such as an increase in the shortness of breath or the swelling of your legs. To help determine if it is safe and appropriate to give these medications, a MUGA scan or echocardiogram is done prior to beginning therapy, specifically with Sutent. This special heart test may be repeated during or after completing treatment.

BLOOD PRESSURE

The systemic agents used for kidney cancer such as immunotherapy, Avastin, Nexavar, Sutent, Afinitor can cause high blood pressure. Your blood pressure will need to be checked on a regular basis while you are on any of these medicines. Whether you are currently taking medication for your blood pressure or not, you may need to work with your oncologist or primary care doctor for treatment of your blood pressure. High-dose Proleukin can cause a severe drop in the blood pressure requiring intensive care monitoring and medications to support the pressure. Although rare (in less than 10 percent), Avastin can cause a lowering of your blood pressure during the infusion. This is a sign of a hypersensitivity reaction, similar to an allergic reaction. You will be given medicine before the infusion to prevent this from happening. If this does occur despite this premedication, your nurse will stop the infusion. Once you have recovered, he or she will resume the infusion, but it will be given slower, over a longer period of time.

INFECTION

Infections develop when your body is not able to fight back and destroy harmful bacteria, viruses, or fungi that enter it. Cancer patients are at high risk of developing an infection because of the cancer itself and the treatments used to fight it. Both can weaken the body's defenses against infection. One way that systemic therapies can cause infection is by decreasing the number of white blood cells in your body (neutropenia). White blood cells fight infection, and when they are too low, it is easy for you to develop a serious infection. Symptoms of infection include spiking a high fever over 100.5°F (38°C), chills, sweating, sore throat, mouth sores, pain or burning during urination, diarrhea, shortness of breath, a productive cough, and swelling redness or pain around an incision or wound are symptoms that an infection may be present. Hand washing or using soapless hand sanitizers is your main defense against infection. You need to be especially cautious around young children who may be carriers of flu viruses, colds, and other respiratory illnesses. Though they can look relatively healthy, young children may be harboring germs. This doesn't mean to stop seeing your children or grandchildren. However, it does mean that you should evaluate how the child is feeling. If the child has any symptoms (runny nose, fever, cough) that would signal to you that this isn't a "healthy" day for them, you may want to keep some distance and not have the child sit on your lap or be close to you. Family members who live with you or people you see frequently should get flu vaccinations to help reduce the risk of unknowingly bringing viruses your way. You don't have to live in isolation, but do be careful about avoiding situations where you could get an infection. Remember you may not have the body's usual defenses because of your disease and treatment. At the first sign you may be getting an infection (fever, cold, etc.), notify your doctor so he or she can evaluate your symptoms and prescribe something for you if indicated.

COGNITIVE DYSFUNCTION

Some refer to this as "chemo brain." People dealing with cancer who are getting systemic therapy as part of their treatment can have trouble remembering names, places, and events or have trouble concentrating or working arithmetic. This is currently an area of scientific study to better understand what is causing it and how to counteract it from happening. If you are finding that these symptoms are severe enough to impact your ability to function well, ask your family to assist you with some tasks that require concentration such as paying bills. Make a list of things you need to do and mark each item off as you do it. Keep your keys in the same place so they are easier to find. Most importantly, get your family members to assist you with medication management. A pill box that has the times of day to take your medications is a good idea rather than relying on your memory. After your systemic therapy is completed, these symptoms usually subside over time.

People who have radiation to the brain for metastatic disease also experience these types of symptoms. In this case, the symptoms are caused by the effects of the radiation on the normal brain tissue causing inflammation. In most cases, these symptoms will improve over time after the radiation treatments have been completed.

It's important to note that some patients who have not had systemic therapy report having these symptoms too. Researchers have therefore been questioning whether part of the problem in memory and with concentration could be related to stress and can be similar to post-traumatic stress syndrome that occurs in response to the stress you may have been experiencing as a result of the cancer diagnosis, treatment, and coping. Remember, you have been going through some very traumatic times: a new cancer diagnosis, cancer surgery, and a future of follow-up evaluations. It is not surprising that even if you haven't had systemic therapy, you can still feel foggy about things as a reaction to the stress.

NAUSEA AND VOMITING

This is a relatively common side effect associated with the administration of some cancer-treatment drugs and radiation (depending on the area of the body that is being irradiated); however, with the development of newer antinausea medicines (called antiemetics), the nausea and vomiting is not as big a problem as it used to be. Pain medications may also cause nausea. If your reaction is severe enough to interfere with eating or drinking, you are likely to become dehydrated. This can be a very serious problem that sometimes requires hospitalization and intravenous fluid infusions. In addition to the antiemetic medicines that your doctor prescribes, changing what you eat and drink may also help control nausea and vomiting. Some specific suggestions include:

- Eat a light meal before each cancer treatment.

- Take small amounts of food and liquids at a time.

- Eat bland foods and liquids.

- Eat dry crackers when you are feeling nauseated.

- Limit the amount of liquids you take with your meals.

- Maintain adequate liquids in between meals; take mostly clear liquids such as water, apple juice, herbal tea, or bouillon.

- Eat cooled foods or foods at room temperature.

- Avoid foods with strong odors.

- Avoid high-fat, greasy, and fried foods.

- Avoid spicy foods, alcohol, and caffeine.

- Suck on ginger or peppermint candies as an additional way to help reduce or prevent nausea.

- Rub peppermint-flavored lip balm above your lip and below your nose so that you are smelling mint as a way to reduce nausea.

- Ask your oncologist for a prescription for an antiemetic and ask if you can take it to prevent, reduce, and control nausea from happening. These medicines include such drugs as Compazine (prochloroperazine), Reglan (metaclopramide), Ansemet (dolasetron), Zofran (ondansetron), Kytril (granisetron), and, on occasion, Ativan (lorazepam).

MOUTH SORES

Also known as mucositis or stomatitis, this is an inflammation of the inside of the mouth and throat and can result in painful ulcers. The painful ulcers are more common with Torisel and Afinitor but can occur with Proleukin and other targeted therapy. Certain medications like steroids that can be given as premedications, or to treat nausea or inflammation in the brain from metastases, may increase the risk of developing an infection in your mouth called thrush or candidiasis. Keep your mouth clean and moist to prevent infection. Brush your teeth with a soft-bristled toothbrush after each meal and rinse regularly. Avoid commercial mouthwashes than contain alcohol because they can irritate the mouth. If you wear dentures that are not fitting properly, you will be more likely to get sores in your mouth from rubbing and irritation. This can be a particular problem if you have experienced or are experiencing weight loss because your gums may shrink, changing the fit of your dentures. See your dentist for an evaluation. If you have dental needs that have not been taken care of prior to starting chemotherapy, ask your oncologist and dentist to talk on the phone and discuss what strategy to use to reduce risk of infection and mouth sores while receiving your treatments. If you are receiving bisphosphonates such as Reclast/Zometa (zolendronic acid), Fosamax (alendronate), or Boniva (ibandronate) to strengthen your bones, be sure to tell your dentist and let your doctor know as well if you need to have oral surgery or tooth extraction.

LOSS OF APPETITE OR TASTE CHANGES

Most of the cancer-therapy drugs can cause a loss of appetite so you just don't feel like eating. You can also experience taste changes in which you have a metallic taste in your mouth or some common eaten foods simply don't taste the same. If you experience this, it is important to try and keep up with your calorie and fluid intake to help maintain your weight and energy. The suggestions listed under the nausea and vomiting section are also helpful if you have loss of appetite or taste changes. Eating small, frequent meals may be easier than sitting down to three big meals a day. Sometimes changing spices may help. If you are having problems maintaining reasonable nutritional intake, ask your doctor or nurse for a consultation with the nutritionist where you are being treated for additional, individualized dietary suggestions.

DIARRHEA

Diarrhea is a common side effect of some of the targeted cancer agents for kidney cancer, such as Sutent or Nexavar. It can also be caused by radiation if you are being treated in the abdominal/back area. If you are having watery, loose stools, some dietary changes may be necessary such as increasing fluid intake, including elements of the "BRAT" diet (bananas, rice, applesauce, and toast) in your meals. However, it is not uncommon to require medication to assist in controlling the diarrhea. Over-the-counter antidiarrhea medicines such as Imodium (loperamide) are often adequate for control of the diarrhea, but there are prescription medications such as Lomotil (diphenoxylate/atropine) are available as well. You should talk to your doctor or nurse if you are experiencing diarrhea.

SKIN RASHES AND EFFECTS

The targeted drugs for kidney cancer can cause a variety of skin problems. Sutent and Nexavar can cause a hand-foot syndrome in which the skin on the palms of the hands and soles of the feet becomes red and inflamed. Painful blistering and peeling can occur. If you develop hand-foot syndrome, check with your doctor or nurse to see if the drug should be stopped until the symptoms improve. Once you recover, it is usually possible to resume treatment with a smaller dose of the medicine. Recently it has been suggested to reduce physical activity in the first 2 weeks of treatment to help prevent or reduce the severity of this syndrome. A variety of rashes can also occur about anywhere on the body, especially from Torisel and radiation therapy. Most are red rashes that may or may not itch. Some are dry and flakey while others have little red bumps that may or may not have some clear drainage. Using moisturizers without perfumes (such as Aveeno products or Lubriderm), minimizing sun exposure, using sunscreens, and wearing long sleeves and a hat may be helpful in preventing or minimizing the skin changes. Cortisone cream, Rash Relief, or Benadryl (diphenhydramine) lotion may be useful in controlling the itching. Talk to your doctor or nurse about specific measures to treat your rash.

Radiation treatments can also cause skin effects that vary in intensity from mild redness to burn-like changes that can be quite uncomfortable. If you experience skin changes from radiation, please discuss these with your radiation doctor or nurse. There are lotions such as Biafine Topical Emulsion that can help relieve the symptoms but some creams and lotions can make the burn worse. Because of this reaction, don't use anything on your skin until you have discussed it with the radiation nurse or doctor!

NEUROLOGICAL PROBLEMS

Some cancer-therapy drugs can cause damage to peripheral nerves. This is referred to as peripheral neuropathy. There are three types of peripheral nerves: sensory, motor, and autonomic. Sensory nerves allow us to feel temperature, pain, vibration, and touch. Motor nerves are responsible for voluntary movement and basically allow us to walk and open doors, for example. Autonomic nerves control involuntary or automatic functions such as breathing, digestion of food, and bowel and bladder activities.

When there is damage to the peripheral nerves, the symptoms depend on the type of peripheral nerves affected. Though cancer-therapy drugs can affect any of the peripheral nerves, the most common ones affected are the sensory nerves causing numbness and tingling in the hands and feet. For patients who already have peripheral neuropathy from other causes (diabetes or excess alcohol, for example), cancer therapy can sometimes make it worse. Symptoms of peripheral neuropathy include:

- Numbness and tingling (which may feel like pins and needles in your hands and/or feet)

- Burning pain in the hands and feet

- Difficulty writing or buttoning a shirt

- Difficulty holding a cup or glass

- Constipation

- Decrease sensation of hot or cold

- Muscle weakness

- Decreased hearing or ringing in the ears (known as tinnitus)

If you develop any of these symptoms, it's important to tell your doctor right away. Describe for him or her the symptoms you are experiencing. If you already have any of these symptoms before starting chemotherapy, make your doctor aware of that as well. Your doctor may decide to prescribe medication for you to take to reduce these symptoms. The medicines most commonly used are drugs that are given to neurology patients for treatment of seizures and depression and may include one or several of the following: Neurontin (gabapentin), Tegretol (carbamazepine), Elavil (amitriptyline), and Lyrica (pregabalin). Some additional measures you should consider taking at home include paying close attention to your walking and avoid having scatter rugs in your house. Keep your home well lit so you can see where you are walking and always wear shoes that fit. If you are still driving a car, be sure you can actually feel the foot pedals. If temperatures are hard to decipher, ask for help in checking the temperature of the bathtub or dishwater as well as any hot beverages you are drinking. Taking care to protect your hands and feet in cold weather is also important because you may not be able to sense the cold.

HAIR LOSS

The technical term is *alopecia* but what patients recognize most clearly is exactly what it is—the hair on your head falls out and if hair on other parts of your body grows rapidly, it may too fall out (such as facial hair, eyelids, or eyebrows). Although targeted drugs for kidney cancer can cause hair loss, more often there is some hair thinning or the hair doesn't seem to be growing at all. Sutent and Nexavar can cause eyebrows and facial hair to turn white. In addition, radiation therapy can also cause hair loss to the area being treated. If you are having radiation to the skull or brain, you should expect to have hair loss.

Hair loss in today's society has become a signal that the person may be a cancer patient. It can be psychologically and physically difficult to cope with thinning hair because it is associated with self-image, sexuality, health status, and other personal issues related to how we feel about ourselves. Discuss with your healthcare team if hair loss or thinning are expected with your regimen. Planning for hair loss such as cutting your hair or getting a wig in advance of hair loss can be helpful so that your hair style, texture, and color can be matched for you. Some insurance companies cover the expense of a wig. Check your policy and see if your insurance company covers "skull prosthesis for side effects of cancer treatment." Costs that are not covered are tax deductible.

There are programs like "Look Good, Feel Good" or "Image Recovery" that most cancer centers or "wellness centers" offer to their patients. These special programs can be helpful to both women and men regarding general appearance, including skin and hair care. They can recommend a variety of help aids and show you how to wear turbans, scarves, hats, and makeup to reduce the obvious appearance, of hair loss. They also have skin care products that can help with skin changes in general. Ask your doctor or nurse if there is a similar program offering at the facility where you are getting your treatment.

If the systemic treatment your doctor is recommending is known to cause hair loss, anticipate this happening usually by the end of your first treatment cycle. Some men and women decide to be proactive and take charge of their hair loss themselves rather than waiting for it to happen. Getting your hair cut short is a good idea or even doing your own buzz cut can be therapeutic since you will control when you lose your hair rather than waiting for the drug to do it. You might consider having a coming-out party for your head. This is a great way for friends and family to participate by bringing you various hats/caps and head coverings.

SEXUAL DYSFUNCTION

The number of people dealing with kidney cancer who are experiencing problems continuing sexual activity isn't clearly known. Even for the general population, sexual dysfunction can be problematic. Some patients can find it very difficult to comfortably discuss this issue with their doctor, though it may be very important to your quality of life. Side effects from your treatment may result in lowering your libido or because of hair loss, weight gain, fatigue, or other symptoms, you simply don't feel well enough to try or confident enough to engage in sexual activity. Physical intimacy is one aspect of a loving relationship. It gives personal pleasure and creates a feeling of closeness to your partner. Sexual intercourse, however, is just one way of being physically intimate. Cuddling, hugging, touching, rubbing, and holding hands are all pleasurable ways to show one another affection. Talk with your partner about your concerns and feelings. This will help both of you to know how to help one another. Experiment with different positions too, finding one that may be more comfortable than another when having sex. If lack of energy impairs your sexual activity, plan ahead for intimacy by identifying when you are feeling higher levels of energy or when you can rest during certain times of the day or week.

Vaginal dryness and erectile dysfunction are common problems as people age and can be made worse with cancer treatments. Vaginal lubricants can help with vaginal dryness. Vaginal discharge, burning, or itching may be signs of a vaginal infection. See your gynecologist if you develop these symptoms so they can be properly treated. If you continue to be sexually active while taking cancer treatments, be sure to use a reliable means of contraception. Many of the cancer treatments can cause birth defects so you want to be sure to prevent pregnancy if this is a possibility. Difficulty with erections can be caused by medications and may improve with agents such as Viagra (sildenfil), Levitra (vardenafil), or Cialis (tadalafil). Work with your doctor to see if they are safe for you with the other medications you are taking.

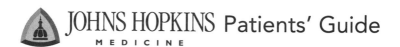

CHAPTER 5

JOHNS HOPKINS Patients' Guide
MEDICINE

STRAIGHT TALK— COMMUNICATION WITH FAMILY, FRIENDS, AND COWORKERS

When you heard the news that you had kidney cancer, you were probably in shock. Stunned. Well, the same things will happen to those who hear the news from you. First, decide whom you need— and want—to tell. Those may be two different groups of people. People you need to tell are those who will be directly affected by it—family members, your boss who needs some information about why and when you will be taking time off from work, and your children, close friends, or others who live with you, all of whom will need to be aware that something very stressful is happening that may change their routines and have an emotional impact on them. There are specialists who can help you in talking about having cancer with children or others, such as social workers and child-life specialists. Ask your doctor or nurse if these specialists are available where you are being treated.

How to tell a child his or her parent has kidney cancer can be tough, no matter what the age of the child. You will need to decide if you and your partner want to tell your children together, if Mom wants to talk to the kids in private, or if Dad will deliver the news. Be honest with your children. They can read you like a book. Conspiracy breeds distrust and will make them more scared than comforted. Explain to them what will be happening in the form of treatment so that they can see you are doing something to get rid of the cancer. Many parents choose to wait to tell their children until after they've seen the doctors and know the treatment plans.

TALKING WITH YOUNG CHILDREN

If your children are little, don't assume they don't know that something significant has happened. Toddlers are especially good at sensing stress and tension in their parents. Though youngsters of this age won't understand what cancer is, they will understand what a boo-boo is so you can tell them that you have a boo-boo that the doctor needs to fix; that sometimes you feel sad about it and other times you are okay. Try to maintain their routine as much as possible.

TALKING WITH TEENS

If your children are older, they may be anxious about how this will impact them—will they get kidney cancer one day too? How will it affect their daily routines? Sometimes teens can be resentful when asked to step in and help out; it simply means that you need to know where they are coming from mentally. You will have to decide who will tell your teens and when, but also how much detail you want to share with them and at what intervals. Remember that teens still need to be teens. Their knowledge base of cancer in general may be to associate it with death. Educate and inform them at their level. Reassure them to the appropriate degree. Tell them that you may need their help with tasks at home for a while but also tell them that you want your treatment to not totally disrupt their lives either. The family as a unit will need to seek a balance of responsibilities.

TELLING PARENTS AND SIBLINGS

Telling your parents is also tough. Parents often wish they had been the ones diagnosed. They want to try to control the situation and can't...and shouldn't. They will need to be given constructive ways to help because no matter what, they will want to help you—even if you feel you don't need it.

Siblings may fear being the next one to be diagnosed in the family. They may need support and information to help them cope with their own anxiety about your diagnosis of kidney cancer. Having them assist with information gathering for you can help engage them in your treatment and empower them with information that will help both of you. Keep your family members informed of how you are doing and how treatment is progressing. Rely on their support. Remember, this is a disease that affects the family. The other family members are also frightened—for you and for themselves.

WHAT TO TELL YOUR BOSS AND COWORKERS

This is tricky. Some people are very open about their illnesses and family crises; others don't utter a word. This is a personal decision. You may choose to tell only a few close friends at work, or you may decide to be very public and take advantage of receiving lots of support. A possible pitfall with telling people is specifically what to tell them and how to ensure that they understood what you said.

The Americans with Disabilities Act provides you with some job protection, so that you are able to work out a schedule with your boss that will meet your medical needs of treatment while ensuring that your work at the office still gets done. You aren't required to tell your boss you have cancer—simply that you are under doctor's care that will require you to miss time from work. Most people, however, will tell their boss that they have been diagnosed with cancer and will be undergoing whatever treatments have been recommended; perhaps saying "kidney cancer surgery" and that additional treatment afterwards may be needed. You are not responsible to provide prognosis information. Again, this is your choice and your personal business.

Telling people initially can be difficult, and it may be difficult to keep these people informed as you move forward with your treatment. You may want to assign someone to be the "information center" and give the announcements about how you are doing, what treatment you are having, pathology results, and so on. Establishing an information contact for people to call for updates and news can help reduce the burden on you and ensure consistency in the information being provided. Email is a good way to make sure that everyone is receiving the same information at the same time and in the same manner, so consider gathering everyone's email addresses and sending out broadcast emails to everyone at once. You will find it a huge timesaver. It also helps prevent family riffs if one family member finds out you called another family member first with the latest update. (Family dynamics escalate during times of stress.)

HOW TO RECRUIT FAMILY AND FRIENDS' SUPPORT

Some friends may avoid calling you after they hear the news. It isn't that they don't care, it's more likely that they don't know what to say, at least without being emotional at the same time. Let them know that even though the diagnosis is upsetting to hear, you need their support. Remember that support from others is part of the treatment plan for you and your family. Other people will ask what they can do to help you so be ready with a list of assignments to delegate. If you haven't already, perhaps one day you will be able to reciprocate and help them in a crisis.

Among the many things they can do include driving the children to school and events, running errands and doing the grocery shopping, making casseroles for your freezer, babysitting, adding you to prayer lists at church, helping with the housework, and—remember, humor builds your immune system—loaning you funny videos to watch or going with you to see a funny movie.

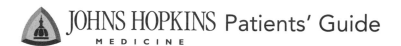

CHAPTER 6

JOHNS HOPKINS Patients' Guide

MEDICINE

MAINTAINING BALANCE—WORK AND LIFE DURING TREATMENT

HOW TO PLAN YOUR CARE AND MINIMIZE DISRUPTIONS IN YOUR LIFE

The last thing you expected to be was the person in your family needing help! You are used to being the one in control, taking care of the family and home, not the one needing care. You are accustomed to juggling busy schedules, functioning as spouse, parent, babysitter, nurse, financial manager, bread winner, counselor, chauffeur, and magician in the family most of the time. For this reason, you might not be good at asking for and accepting help from others. Your kidney cancer treatment may alter roles, play havoc with schedules, and create additional stress including financial concerns for you, family members, and friends helping during this time. It is inevitable, but it can be managed.

Patients with children especially may experience a variety of role changes. Your spouse may be putting young children to bed because you don't feel well at night. Older children may be asked to help with meal preparation, yard work, or laundry. It's important for you and your family to talk about your schedules and how treatment needs will impact them. Design a new schedule to best meet your needs and those of your loved ones—with as little change as possible.

This is also the time to ask for—and accept—help from other family members, neighbors, and friends. After all, one day they may need your help in a similar way.

Try to maintain your children's routines as much as possible. Change creates stress no matter what the age; even an infant who is fed an hour later than usual expresses his/her opinions about the altered schedule. Let your children know in advance if there will be a change in their routine. Keep children informed about what is happening related to your treatment. Encourage them to help and play an active role in the treatment, too. You might consider having younger children (ages 6–12) go with you to the hospital if you are getting one of your chemo treatments to better understand what is happening. Ask them how they picture the chemotherapy traveling through your veins destroying any bad cells that might be lingering. Have them draw pictures to cheer you up. They can open the get-well cards you receive in the mail too. Explain why you don't feel well and the importance of playing quietly on certain days after treatment. Let young children know that they can't catch kidney cancer and also aren't in any way the cause of it either.

HELPFUL HINTS

To help prepare for surgery, request to meet with a nurse for some preoperative instruction. Your surgeon may arrange this for you. You will want to know in advance how long you will be out of commission from doing your routine activities, what clothing will be best to wear following your surgery, when you will be allowed to resume driving, go back to work, and so forth.

If you are scheduled to have systemic therapy, make a chart of when your treatments will be or when you will need to see the doctor and when you will need blood tests done. See about having appointments for treatments toward the end of the week so you can have the weekend to rest up (when hopefully there will be additional help around the house available to you). Decide if you want someone to go with you for the intravenous treatments. You will need someone to drive you and pick you up for at least the first cycle of treatments because you may be given premedications that may make you drowsy. You may be in the chemotherapy infusion center for several hours, so plan accordingly. The day needs to be as laid back as possible for you. Depending on who is available to help and what your schedules end up being, you or your spouse/partner may decide chemo days are "pizza nights" for the kids or the time to pull out the casserole your neighbor made from the freezer.

If hair loss is a potential side effect, it usually begins around 3 weeks after you start treatment. If you want to be proactive, consider cutting your hair short or even doing a buzz cut prior to your hair falling out on its own. Friends and family can supply you with various head coverings—baseball caps, turbans, hats, and the like. Your kids may want to make you some funny ones to wear around your home.

For radiation, consider the timing of the treatments. Some people prefer to schedule it at the very beginning or the end of the day while others schedule the treatment around their lunch break. Since this treatment is daily, you will want it to cause as little disruption to your daily routine as possible. Most radiation facilities have patients in and out in under 30 minutes. You spend more time getting your clothes off and on than you do actually getting your treatment.

CONTINUING WORK

Most men and women return to work after recovering from their kidney cancer surgery. If systemic therapy is needed, many are still able to continue to work. Time missed from work can be minimized if planned out; however, your employer should know that you may be less reliable because of fatigue or other side effects. It actually is to your advantage to continue to work because stopping work can be an additional stressor for you with the resulting change in income, not to mention that it abruptly changes your routine. You want to continue to feel productive, be surrounded by supportive coworkers, and not be spending every waking moment thinking about cancer. Sit down with your supervisor and plan out a schedule that works for both of you. There may be some times when you work only half a day because you are getting chemotherapy in the afternoon, then taking off the following day. During radiation, you may be coming in an hour later to work or leaving 30 minutes early to get to your daily radiation appointment. Employers know the importance of being flexible, and you are protected to some degree by the Family Medical Leave Act (FMLA) that entitles you and your spouse to time off for appointments. You should talk to your human resources department about this option. If you work around small children (especially those of toddler age), this may be problematic particularly if you experience changes in your blood counts that would put you at greater risk of getting a serious infection. A great deal will depend on how you are feeling when you need to begin systemic treatment. Do not feel like a failure if you don't feel able to work. You are going through many changes and stresses and may need to be off of work to recover. If you are staying home from work, check with your employer about FMLA, and short- and long-term disability options. A social worker may help you investigate these options as well.

Remember, that despite the best-laid plans, things can happen that will disrupt or negate them. It doesn't mean, however, that you or your family and/or support people have failed. It simply means that you and your family and/or support people need to be flexible in order to help you through this time of changes to you, your body, your relationships, and your work.

WHEN I MIGHT EXPECT NOT TO FEEL WELL

There are potential side-effects associated with any treatment. Usually if you are going to have gastrointestinal (GI) side effects such as diarrhea or nausea and vomiting, it will be 16–48 hours after the completion of the anticancer drug infusion. For oral drugs, nausea may occur at almost any time after taking the pill. However, nausea can also be something that slowly builds over time. Request a prescription for antinausea medicines in advance so you can also head off nausea and vomiting symptoms before they get too bad.

Other side effects with the targeted therapy may get worse as the treatment continues. For instance, fatigue and diarrhea from Sutent may not be a problem until the second or third week and then gets better and goes away during the time off of the drug.

Not everyone will need to have radiation. If it is recommended for you to take radiation, anticipate feeling fine until about the last 2 weeks or so. At this point in time you may notice increased fatigue. This is because radiation effects are cumulative. Give yourself extra time to rest at night and even take a catnap in the middle of the day if possible. Remember that other side effects will depend on the part of your body that is being treated. Talk to your radiation doctor or nurse about what to expect.

INFECTION PREVENTION

Anticipate that on certain days your white blood cells will go down in response to having received systemic therapy. These are the days when you are more vulnerable to getting a cold, flu, or other forms of infection. You will want to be careful when in the presence of children, because they can be infectious even though they may not act like they are sick. Wearing a mask is beneficial if you can't avoid being around them in a closed environment. Frequent hand washing with soap or soapless sanitizers is the main thing that everyone, including you, can do to help prevent infections. Try to maintain a balanced diet; one that is rich in washed fruits and vegetables helps to improve your immune system and resistance.

See your dentist to have your teeth cleaned and for any dental work that needs to be done before you start therapy to prevent any later problems related to tooth infections. Systemic therapy doesn't cause dental problems but if one is brewing, it can make it worse due to your immune system being taxed and unable to fight infection as well as it did before.

Getting a flu shot before you start therapy is advisable too. Depending on the time of year that you are being treated, getting one early in the flu season, then another one later in the season may help maintain your defense. If you need to travel by air while undergoing therapy and your white blood counts are low, you may want to wear a mask to reduce your risk of exposure to infections. Your mission is to try to be as healthy as possible during your treatments and reduce your risk of exposure to infection as much as possible. The nurse who is working with you during your treatments can mark on your chart the days when you will be particularly vulnerable to infection. In addition, your blood will be drawn periodically to see what effects the therapy has had on your bone marrow and body chemistry.

Remember there are people that can help you with planning and coping with the changes in your life. Don't be afraid to ask for help from the many professionals available to you such as a social worker, chaplain, or counselor if the road gets bumpy. Your doctor or nurse can help you make the initial contact.

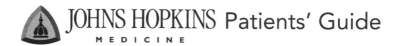

CHAPTER 7

JOHNS HOPKINS Patients' Guide
MEDICINE

Surviving Kidney Cancer— Re-engaging in Mind and Body Health After Treatment

SURVIVORSHIP

When do you consider yourself a survivor? The most common definition is that the moment you are diagnosed—whether you have chosen treatment or not—you are a survivor. Some people, however, don't consider themselves survivors until treatment is completed. There are thousands of people who are kidney cancer survivors. You are among an elite group. After your surgery and finishing any additional treatment, however, rather than feeling like celebrating, you may feel like you fell off a cliff. Not an unusual reaction either. You've been so focused on actively fighting this disease that when the treatment is over, you feel a sense of letdown—fear, too, that you haven't done enough or that there isn't additional treatment to continue to take as a means of preventing recurrence. Fear of recurrence remains the biggest issue that survivors have to deal with today. Although many people will not have to face a recurrence of this disease, it can be hard to learn to trust your body again. You may become a "body watcher"—wondering if new aches or pains or other symptoms mean the cancer is back. Staying in the know about the latest research that has been published about kidney cancer can be helpful and empowering. Taking measures to help yourself regain an emotional balance is wise too. Some cancer centers offer special survivor retreats or celebrations for this purpose. But at the very least, you and your oncologist should have a plan that includes the follow-up schedule (how often and what testing is involved), further risk education related to your kidney cancer, cancer screening for other cancers, general health assessment, etc. There should be a partnership between you, your cancer doctors, and your primary care doctor.

COUNSELING

If your doctor or nurse recommends that you consider seeing a counselor, don't feel like you have failed at getting yourself back on track. It's hard. Many people benefit from seeing a therapist posttreatment to help them re-engage in their lives physically and emotionally healthier. Sometimes we simply need a professional sounding board to hear our hidden thoughts and fears and help us gain perspective about what and what not to worry about. You want to regain control over your life. This can take assistance from others who are professionally trained at doing this. The diagnosis and treatment of kidney cancer is life altering. There is no operator's manual for this experience. Talk with other survivors, too, to help you realize that what you are experiencing is the norm and not the exception.

MANAGING THE LONG-TERM SIDE EFFECTS OF TREATMENT

It would be great if at the time that treatment ended, all the side effects associated with it ended too, but this is not the case. You may be dealing with residual side effects of incisional pain, peripheral neuropathy, difficulty concentrating, fatigue, night sweats, or other unpleasantness. Give your body time to heal and adjust. Some side effects like fatigue can linger for up to a year, particularly if you had additional treatment after your surgery. Don't expect to feel back to yourself right away. There is a period of psychological and physical adjustment. Your body needs time. Allow it this time for recovery. (See **Chapter 4** for the management of side effects.)

LIVING A HEALTHIER LIFESTYLE

Taking charge of your health and psychological well-being should be a priority for you now. Here are some helpful ways to accomplish this and feel good doing it.

NUTRITION

If you eat healthier, and watch your weight, you may help to reduce your risk of recurrence of this disease. Doctors know that high-fat diets that encourage packing on the pounds can increase risk due to the additional weight gain. Eating a diet rich in green and orange vegetables is smart for your health as well as your heart. This doesn't mean that you have to give up chocolate nut sundaes for the rest of your life. Eat smart. Save high-fat and high-calorie foods for special times and rewards—just don't make them part of your daily life. If you have had your kidney removed, you may be told to avoid a high-protein diet, as this may be harmful to your remaining kidney. But your body needs protein for health maintenance—so remember, everything in moderation! Heart-healthy menus are also cancer-healthy menus.

EXERCISE

Exercising is another way to help reduce the risk of recurrence. This doesn't mean you need to become a marathon runner and press 400 pounds at the gym, but it does mean finding an exercise program that works for you, that you can commit to, and that makes you feel good. If you enjoy an exercise program, it is in an environment that makes you feel comfortable, you feel better after you do it, and it is something you are able to stick with, then it's a winner for you. Power walking is one option to consider. Walking three times a week for an hour will suffice. Working out at the gym three times a week also will. Exercising with a friend usually makes it more enjoyable and helps you to stick to it, because you have a buddy rooting you on.

STRESS

Emotional turmoil affects your immune system and your immune system needs to be in good shape to fight cancer cells and prevent them from growing. Though it's a nice fantasy to picture yourself sitting on a beach reading a book, worry free, this isn't reality. You will be expected to resume your chaotic life, including family responsibilities and work duties. Reassessing how you react to stressful situations is something you can do, however. Kidney cancer can teach us that we really don't have to sweat the small stuff. Making time for you is important, including after your treatment is completed. Put things into perspective before reacting to them. Is it really a crisis that your mother-in-law came over and you haven't dusted or vacuumed the floors? Or that your boss gave you a big project to do just as you were beginning to bounce back from surgery? You have been through much bigger and more significant stuff. Learn deep breathing techniques, meditation, yoga, or other forms of relaxation therapy. They can be helpful to you in reducing stress and keeping life in perspective.

AVOID SMOKE AND ALCOHOL

Avoid smoke, including secondary smoke. If you smoke, you should try to quit if you haven't already begun to do so. Cigarette smoking affects all of the cells in your body—not just the lungs, mouth, and throat. If you have friends who smoke, remind them that if they care about you, they will take their cigarettes outside. This includes other people who live with you. If they refuse and still smoke around you, then they aren't your friends. Also, limit alcohol to one drink a day if you are a woman and two if you are a man. And remember, wine is possibly better than hard liquor or beer.

SETTING NEW GOALS

You have just completed treatment that was life altering. You have perhaps stared death in the face and survived what you thought wasn't possible to overcome. This is an ideal time to step back and reassess your life, looking at how you want to leave your mark on this earth, and realizing you are going to be around to make that mark. Some people decide they want to go back to school or launch a new career.

Others decide they want to work part time rather than full time, investigate other types of work, or retire and spend more time with their loved ones. It's your call. It's your life. Consider setting short- and long-term goals. Some goals may be directed at living a healthier lifestyle; others may be focused on how you want to make a difference for others who come behind you. Join alliances to make a difference or strike out on your own regarding how you want to spend the rest of your life. What you thought was important before may have different meaning to you now. This shift in attitude can be quite confusing, though, to those around you who were expecting things to return to "normal." You need to find your "new normal," and let your family and friends know that you are working hard to accomplish this. This experience has changed you—hopefully for the better—and life will be considered more precious and valued than it was before. You have been faced with your own mortality. Communicate your thoughts with your family and friends. Keep a journal to record them. Journaling can be very therapeutic and may be a special part of your legacy.

SEEING THE WORLD THROUGH DIFFERENT EYES

It can be hard for people you spend time with—family, friends, and coworkers—to understand that you are not quite the same person you were before your diagnosis. Hopefully, you are different in all the right ways: mindful of how precious life is, never taking anything for granted, valuing relationships differently perhaps than you did before. Consider getting involved as a volunteer. One of the best ways to move forward with your experience with cancer is to help those who are diagnosed after you. By helping someone else, you help yourself psychologically, because although recovery from kidney cancer itself may take a finite time physically, emotional recovery can take a lifetime. It can be, and usually is, life altering in a positive way. Consider volunteering where you received your surgery or treatments. Let your doctor know that you would be happy to talk to another person who is facing surgery or systemic treatment for kidney cancer. Volunteer for a kidney cancer organization or a general cancer organization such as the American Cancer Society that has a chapter in your area. This can be very rewarding and is a great way to give back as well as help others and yourself. Educate others and help promote kidney cancer awareness in your local community.

CHAPTER 8

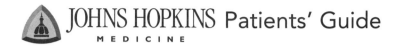

MANAGING RISK—WHAT IF MY CANCER COMES BACK?

The risk of recurrence remains one of the most feared issues that people deal with when they are diagnosed and particularly when they have finished their initial cancer treatment. Learning what to look for, when, how, and for how long is helpful. Putting the risk of recurrence into perspective is extremely important to your psychological well-being. People who have undergone nephrectomy and who had the disease in an early stage, in general, have a risk of recurrence of about 10 to 30 percent. Prognostic factors such as stage and grade of the tumor and if it was confined to the kidney will influence your specific risk. In general, however, the risk of recurrence is relatively low for those diagnosed with early-stage kidney cancer. For people who are diagnosed with the disease in a later stage such as stage 3 or 4, the risk of recurrence increases to 40 to 60 percent. The period of time that the risk of recurrence is greatest is during the first 2 years. It then diminishes over the next 3 years until the 5-year mark when most cancer survivors feel they have been cured. However, even when the 5-year mark is reached, the risk of recurrence never becomes zero. Continued follow-up and monitoring is important in order to discover a recurrence early.

PREVENTION AND MONITORING FOR RECURRENCE

If the cancer has been completely removed, a CAT scan of the chest and abdomen is recommended 4 to 6 months after the surgery as a baseline. Scans are then repeated at regular intervals. During the first 2 years, CAT scans of the chest, abdomen, and pelvis or CAT scans of the abdomen and pelvis with chest X-rays may be done more frequently (up to two to four times a year depending on the stage of the cancer) to look for any recurrence. If everything continues to remain negative, the scans may be decreased to one to two times a year until the 5-year mark. It is also important for you to report symptoms that don't go away in 1 to 2 weeks or any that get progressively worse. These might include pain, increasing shortness of breath, a cough, a loss in appetite or weight, or night sweats. New symptoms that don't go away and get progressively worse can mean that the cancer is showing up again. Although not all symptoms like these mean that the cancer is back or growing, it is important to inform your oncologist of any symptoms so that they can be evaluated. Wherever the cancer might show up again—in the lungs, bone, liver, or brain, it is still considered kidney cancer and not a new cancer such as brain cancer or lung cancer. Because of this, it will be treated with therapies approved or being studied for kidney cancer.

TREATMENT OPTIONS (LOCAL VERSUS DISTANT RECURRENCE)

When the cancer comes back, there are a variety of treatment options depending on the location of the recurrences. Sometimes a single metastatic site in the lung or in the area where the kidney was removed can be surgically removed, but that doesn't prevent other sites from showing up. However, a small single recurrent lesion might be managed effectively with removal.

In general, if your cancer comes back, that is the time to start systemic therapy such as Proleukin or one of the targeted drugs (Sutent, Nexavar, Torisel, or Afinitor). If you are physically well, with excellent heart, liver, and kidney function, and your cancer has spread only to your lungs, you may be a candidate for high-dose Proleukin therapy. That therapy requires hospitalization and potentially intensive care for about 7 to 10 days and is repeated several times if you can tolerate it. If the cancer responds and goes away, the long-term survival outlook is excellent. If the cancer has come back in multiple places or there is a large amount of cancer to treat, the systemic, targeted drugs would be recommended usually starting with Sutent or Nexavar. The goal of the targeted therapies is to keep the disease under control. Although the cancer may shrink while on these agents, some of these drugs show a modest increase in long-term survival.

Depending on the location of the recurrence, another option may be radiation. If it is in the bone, then radiation is used to treat the area affected by the cancer. Depending on the severity of the bone lesion, surgery may also be employed to stabilize the bone structure. Bisphophonates, such as Reclast/Zometa, may be used for metastatic disease to the bone in an effort to help reduce bone fracture or other bone involvement. Radiation can also be used alone or with surgery to treat the cancer that has come back in the brain. Cryoablation or radiofrequency ablation may be employed for isolated lesions of recurrence.

Because it is unlikely for the therapies that are currently available to be curative once the cancer comes back or has spread, doctors are always trying to find new and better ways to treat kidney cancer. If your cancer does come back, you may be offered a clinical trial of a new drug or approach to treatment that is being tested in people with kidney cancer. This could be a phase III study where a new kidney cancer drug is being tested against a standard kidney cancer drug or a phase 2 study where a new drug is being tested to see how effective it is against kidney cancer. There may also be phase 1 studies for which you could qualify where the drug is either being tested for the first time in humans or is being tested for the first time in a new combination. (See **Chapter 3** for more details about types of clinical trials.)

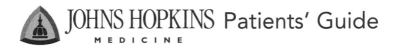

CHAPTER 9

JOHNS HOPKINS Patients' Guide
MEDICINE

My Cancer Isn't Curable— What Now?

UNDERSTANDING GOALS OF TREATMENT FOR METASTATIC DISEASE

It can be devastating to hear that your disease has come back or has spread to other parts of your body. When this happens, the goals of the treatment plan change from one of cure to one of control of the disease. The goal is to control the disease and its symptoms so that you can maintain your quality of life for as long as possible. It can be a challenge to balance treatment with quality of life because all treatments have side effects. If you have just learned that your kidney cancer has spread, you may opt for treatment now or delay for a period of time to see the pace of the disease. If your kidney cancer isn't growing or is growing slowly, you may choose to continue ongoing monitoring with regular scans as long as you do not have any symptoms of the disease. Because the targeted therapies do not always cause a reduction in the size of the cancer, beginning therapy when the cancer is not growing may simply give you side effects without changing your cancer.

Your cancer will now be treated more like a chronic condition such as hypertension or diabetes that requires ongoing evaluation and management. Sometimes everything is stable and not changing, so no change in treatment or monitoring is required. However, if something changes such as developing a new site of kidney cancer or unacceptable side effects of the current treatment, then the approach to management may need to be modified. Thus, ongoing evaluations for the treatment and the control of metastatic kidney cancer are required. Faced with the reality that your cancer isn't curable at this point, you may wish to think about how this changes your goals as you move forward.

SETTING SHORT-TERM GOALS

It may not be unreasonable to have some long-term goals, but you may be disappointed when you can't achieve them. Instead, it may be better to set short-term goals from one milestone to another; to see how the cancer responds to the recommended treatment, to see how well you can tolerate the treatment. Short-term goals may be 6 months to a year in length. Are there people who have lived for years with metastatic disease? Yes, but unfortunately, they are not the majority. Discuss what to expect with your doctor. Be hopeful; be optimistic but realistic. Doing something that is important to you may need to be done sooner than originally planned. The goal may be for you to be here in 3 years but first see how your body responds to treatment of the metastasis before making any long-term plans or goals. Ask your doctor how long you will be taking a treatment before scans will be repeated to see how effective the medications are in stabilizing or shrinking the cancer. Find out when in the treatment schedule you would be able to do things like travel or other activities. It is important that you keep on living and doing the things that you want or need to do for yourself or your family and friends.

QUALITY OF LIFE VERSUS QUANTITY OF LIFE

The goal for anyone should be to maintain a good quality of life and not simply focus on how many days, weeks, or years you are here. Quantity may not be as important now as quality of life. Living a long time in severe pain, unable to take care of your daily needs, and not enjoying life is probably not the way you would want to live. A shorter length of time during which you feel pretty good and are enjoying family and friends may be far better than a longer length of time when you have severe symptoms and are unable to do the things that give you pleasure. If you are experiencing a great deal of pain, you need to let your doctor or nurse know! There are medications to control pain. The doctors and nurses may not know that you are suffering if you don't tell them. Sometimes patients are frightened about reporting new symptoms, fearing they will hear that this means the prognosis is worse. Although that may be true, you may also be able to have radiation or other approaches that will make you feel better and help you live better. You must let your doctor and nurse know how you are feeling so that appropriate interventions can be undertaken.

WHEN SHOULD I STOP TREATMENT

This is not an easy question to ask your doctor and not an easy question for him or her to answer either. Still, having a candid discussion about stopping treatment is very valu-able. It may require you meeting with your doctor one on one when your family isn't accompanying you. It may be easier to talk frankly without your spouse, child, or parent sitting beside you since they may not want to hear the an-swer to this question. However, it is important for you and your family to know what to expect and how best to help you when things aren't going well. In general, treatment can continue as long as you are responding without severe side effects, there are treatment options to offer you, and your quality of life is being maintained. Ultimately, though, it is your choice whether to continue. There may come a time, however, when your doctor does not recommend ad-ditional treatment for your cancer—often because you may be too sick to tolerate additional treatment or the treatment is no longer helping you.

You want your doctor to be very honest and open with you—to tell you when he or she recommends stopping treat-ment. That being said, just because your doctor does not recommend additional therapy or you decide to stop, you will still be taken care of; your doctor and nurse will still try to help you maintain as much quality of life and control your symptoms as possible. Being prepared for such a time can be helpful. This means asking your doctor how long he or she anticipates being able to treat your cancer, what drugs are available for you now and in the future, and what clinical trials may be available to you.

It is always a good idea to have your affairs in order and your wishes known. There is a tendency to postpone do-ing this, perhaps because you don't want to think about it; if you don't think about it, it won't happen. Still, you know that that is not the case. Everyone ultimately has to face the end of life so it is important to have personal, financial, and medical affairs in order. Life can be very unpredictable. Fatal accidents or heart attacks happen. You are in a situation that provides you with some insight into your future and what the future may hold for you. Take advantage of this insight and make sure you have a will, an advanced directive, that your finances in order, and that your personal wishes are clearly known to your next of kin or person who will have your medical power of attorney if you are not able to speak for yourself.

HOSPICE/PALLIATIVE CARE

When you are approaching the end of life, there are special medical services available to help you and those closest to you in this stage of life. Palliative care and hospice care are approaches that focus on you and maintaining your quality of life—actively treating your physical symptoms as well as psychological and spiritual concerns—and ultimately assisting you and those closest to you with bereavement. The goals of palliative care are to help with personal care and symptom control and to maintain a good quality of life. You can continue with some ongoing treatment of your cancer and also receive additional support. Hospice is a program that can also help during this time—to help you and those closest to you with your personal care, symptom control, and spiritual and psychological care; to help maintain some quality of life; and to help you to say good-bye to family and friends. Hospice also assists your loved ones with bereavement after you are gone. A referral from your doctor is needed for hospice and commonly is arranged around the time the decision is made that treatment is no longer benefitting you. Hospice care can be provided in a hospice facility or in the home. It's your choice. Again, your quality of life is paramount. Honoring your wishes and spending time as you want to spend it is the mission now. Counseling is provided to you and family members and spiritual needs are addressed for everyone. This is your time with family and friends; this is your time for reflection and to gain a sense of peace.

Talk to your oncology doctor or nurse about these programs/approaches to care. Sometimes talking about them earlier in your disease can give you the information that will be helpful while you are still receiving treatment. It can help you and your family and friends to be prepared for what may lie ahead.

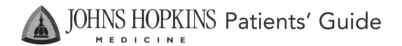

CHAPTER 10

JOHNS HOPKINS Patients' Guide

MEDICINE

KIDNEY CANCER
IN OLDER ADULTS
BY GARY SHAPIRO, MD

Sixty-five is the average age that people develop kidney cancer, but its frequency is increasing as the population ages, especially in men. In the next 25 years, the number of people who are 65 years of age and older will double, and the largest increases in cancer incidence will occur in those older than 80 years of age.

Older adults with cancer often have other chronic health problems and may be taking multiple medications that can affect their cancer treatment plan. Prejudice, misunderstanding, and limited access to clinical trials often prevent older patients from getting the timely cancer treatment that they need.

Older men and woman may not have adequate screening for kidney cancer and when a cancer is found, it is too often ignored or undertreated. As a result, older individuals often have more advanced stage cancer and worse outcomes than younger patients.

WHY IS THERE MORE CANCER IN OLDER PEOPLE?

The organs in our body are made up of cells. Cells divide and multiply as the body needs them. Cancer develops when cells in a part of the body grow out of control. The body has a number of ways of repairing damaged control mechanisms, but as we get older, these do not work as well. Although current healthier lifestyles allow us to avoid death from infection, heart attack, and stroke, we may now live long enough for a cancer to develop. People who live longer have increased exposure to cancer-causing agents (carcinogens) in the environment (like tobacco, asbestos, cadmium, and other workplace substances). They are also more likely to be overweight or have kidney diseases that increase the risk for developing kidney cancer. Aging decreases the body's ability to protect us from carcinogens and to repair cells that are damaged by these and other processes.

DECISION MAKING: 7 PRACTICAL STEPS

1. GET A DIAGNOSIS

No matter how "typical" the signs and symptoms, first impressions are sometimes wrong. Sometimes malignant kidney tumors are due to a lymphoma, urothelial (transitional cell), or some other type of cancer that behaves, and is treated, very differently than renal-cell kidney cancer. It might even be benign. That blood in your urine may be a simple infection or the suspicious mass on your CAT scan may be a nonmalignant cyst. A diagnosis helps you and your family understand what to expect and how to prepare for the future, even if you cannot get curative treatment. Knowing the diagnosis also helps your doctor treat your symptoms better. Many people find "not knowing" very hard, and are relieved when they finally have an explanation for their symptoms. Sometimes a frail patient is obviously dying, and diagnostic studies can be an additional burden. In such cases, it may be quite reasonable to focus on symptom relief (palliation) without knowing the details of the diagnosis.

2. KNOW THE CANCER'S STAGE

The cancer's stage defines your prognosis and treatment options. No one can make informed decisions without it. Just as there may be times when the burdens of diagnostic studies may be too great, it may also be appropriate to do without full staging in a very frail, dying patient.

As it is in younger patients, the stage is determined by the size of the tumor, the presence or absence of cancer in lymph nodes, or its spread (metastasis) to other organs. When doctors combine this with information regarding how far the cancer has grown into the veins that come out of your kidney, they can predict what impact, if any, your kidney cancer is likely to have on your life expectancy and quality of life.

3. KNOW YOUR LIFE EXPECTANCY

Anticancer treatment should be considered if you are likely to live long enough to experience symptoms or premature death from kidney cancer. If your life expectancy is so short that the cancer will not significantly affect it, there may be no reason to treat your cancer.

However, chronological age (how old you are) should not be the only thing that decides how your cancer should, or should not, be treated. Despite advanced age, people who are relatively well often have a life expectancy that is longer than their life expectancy with kidney cancer. The average 70-year-old woman is likely to live another 16 years, and the average 70-year-old man another 12 years. A similar 85-year-old can expect to live an additional 5 to 6 years, and remain independent for most of that time. Even an unhealthy 75-year-old man or woman probably will live 5 to 6 more years, long enough to suffer symptoms and early death from recurrent kidney cancer.

4. UNDERSTAND THE GOALS

The Goals of Treatment

It is important to be clear whether the goal of treatment is cure (surgery, radiation therapy, or both combined, for early stage kidney cancer) or palliation (radiation or systemic therapy for incurable locally advanced or metastatic kidney cancer). If the goal is palliation, you need to understand if the treatment plan will extend your life, control your symptoms, or both. How likely is it to achieve these goals, and how long will you enjoy its benefits?

When the goal of treatment is palliation, systemic therapy should never be administered without defined endpoints and timelines. It should be clear to everyone what "counts" as success, how it will be determined (for example, a symptom controlled or a smaller mass on a CAT scan), and when. You and your family should understand what your options are at each step, and how likely each is to meet your goals. If this is not clear, ask your doctor to explain it in words that you understand.

The Goals of the Patient

In addition to the traditional goals of tumor response, increased survival, and symptom control, older cancer patients often have goals related to quality of life. These may include physical and intellectual independence, spending quality time with your family, taking trips, staying out of the hospital, or even economic stability. At times, palliative care or hospice may meet these goals better than active anticancer treatment. In addition to the medical team, older patients often turn to family, friends, and clergy to help guide them.

5. DETERMINE IF YOU ARE FIT OR FRAIL

Deciding how to treat cancer in someone who is older requires a thorough understanding of her general health and social situation. Decisions about cancer treatment should never focus on age alone.

Age Is Not a Number

Your actual age (chronological age) has limited influence on how cancer will respond to therapy or its prognosis. Biological and other changes associated with aging are more reliable in estimating an individual's vigor, life expectancy, or the risk of treatment complications. These changes include malnutrition, loss of muscle mass and strength, depression, dementia, falls, social isolation, and the ability to accomplish daily activities such as dressing, bathing, eating, shopping, housekeeping, and managing one's finances or medication.

Chronic Illnesses

Older cancer patients are likely to have chronic illnesses (comorbidity) that affect their life expectancy; the more that you have, the greater the effect. This effect has very little impact on the behavior of the cancer itself, but studies show that comorbidity has a major impact on treatment outcome and its side effects.

6. BALANCE BENEFITS AND HARMS

Fit older kidney cancer patients respond to treatment similarly to their younger counterparts. However, a word of caution is in order. Until recently, few studies included older individuals, and it may not be appropriate to apply these findings to the diverse group of older cancer patients.

The side effects of cancer treatment are never less in the elderly. In addition to the standard side effects, there are significant age-related toxicities to consider. Though most of these are more a function of frailty than chronological age, even the fittest senior cannot avoid the physical effects of aging. In addition to the changes in fat and muscle that you see in the mirror, there are age-related changes in your kidney, liver, and digestive (gastrointestinal) function. These changes affect how your body absorbs and metabolizes anticancer drugs and other medicines. The average senior takes many different medicines (to control, for example, high blood pressure, high cholesterol, osteoporosis, diabetes, arthritis, etc.). This "polypharmacy" can cause undesirable side effects as the many drugs interact with each other and the anticancer medications.

7. GET INVOLVED

Healthcare providers and family members often underestimate the physical and mental abilities of older people and their willingness to face chronic and life-threatening conditions. Studies clearly show that older patients want detailed and easily understood information about potential treatments and alternatives. Patients and families may consider cancer untreatable in the aged, and not understand the possibilities offered by treatment.

Although patients with dementia pose a unique challenge, they are frequently capable of participating in goal setting and simple discussions about treatment side effects and logistics. Caring family members and friends are often able to share the patient's life story so that healthcare workers can work with them to make decisions consistent with the patient's values and desires. This of course is no substitute for a well-thought-out and properly executed living will or healthcare proxy.

While it is hard to face the possibility of life-threatening events at any age, it is always better to be prepared and to "put your affairs in order." In addition to estate planning and wills, it is critical that you outline your wishes regarding medical care at the end of life, and make legal provisions for someone to make those decisions if you are unable to make them for yourself.

TREATING KIDNEY CANCER

YOU NEED A TEAM

Cancer care changes rapidly, and it is hard for the generalist to keep up to date, so referral to a specialist is essential. The needs of an older cancer patient often extend beyond the doctor's office and the traditional services provided by visiting nurses. These needs may include transportation, nutrition, and emotional, financial, physical, or spiritual support. When an older woman or man with kidney cancer is the primary caregiver for a frail or ill spouse, grandchildren, or other family members, special attention is necessary to provide for their needs as well. Older cancer patients cared for in geriatric oncology programs benefit from multidisciplinary teams of oncologists, geriatricians, psychiatrists, pharmacists, physiatrists, social workers, nurses, clergy, and dieticians, all working together as a team to identify and manage the stressors that can limit effective cancer treatment.

SURGERY

Surgery is the standard of care for most early stage cancers of the kidney (see **Chapter 3**), regardless of age. Like other treatment options, surgery in some older individuals may involve risks related to decreases in body organ function (especially the heart and lung), and it is essential that the surgeon and anesthetist work closely with your primary care physician (or a consultant) to fully assess and treat these problems before, during, and after the operation.

Surgery is as effective in elderly patients as in younger patients, but it does have a higher rate of complications (including death) in older individuals who have other medical problems (comorbidities). Because these complications are also related to the amount of blood lost during the operation, the time spent in surgery, and the total numbers of days spent in the hospital, minimally invasive surgery techniques are particularly attractive in treating older patients. When possible, older patients with kidney cancer should consider laparoscopic nephrectomy and partial nephrectomy. Cryoablation, radiofrequency ablation, and arterial embolization are particularly appealing in frail individuals or those with a very high surgical risk.

RADIATION THERAPY

Radiation therapy is rarely the treatment of choice for early stage cancer of the kidney.

Radiation therapy usually provides excellent symptom relief (palliation) in metastatic and other incurable situations. It is particularly effective in treating pain caused by kidney cancer metastases to the bone. A short course of radiation therapy often allows patients with advanced cancer to lower (or even eliminate) their dose of opioid (narcotic) pain relievers. Although these medicines do an excellent job of controlling pain, they often cause confusion, falls, and constipation in older patients. Thus, even hospice patients suffering from localized metastatic bone pain should consider the option of palliative radiation therapy.

The fatigue that usually accompanies radiation therapy can be quite profound in the elderly, even in those who are fit. Often the logistical details (like daily travel to the hospital for a 6-week course of treatment) are the hardest for older people. It is important that you discuss these potential problems with your family and social worker prior to starting radiation therapy.

SYSTEMIC THERAPY

Renal-cell cancer usually does not respond to traditional cytotoxic chemotherapy (Gemzar, Xeloda, Adrucil), but newer targeted treatments (Sutent, Nexavar, Torisel, Afinitor), are more effective. Though they may temporarily control advanced kidney cancer, they are no substitute for surgical techniques in potentially curable kidney cancer.

Nonfrail older cancer patients respond to targeted therapy (see **Chapter 3**) similarly to their younger counterparts. Reducing the dose of chemotherapy based purely on chronological age may seriously affect the effectiveness of treatment. Managing chemotherapy-associated toxicity with appropriate supportive care is crucial in the elderly population to give them the best chance of cure and survival or to provide the best palliation.

Although targeted therapy is generally well tolerated in the elderly, cytokine therapy (Intron A/Roferon A or Proleukin) is particularly toxic for the majority of older patients, especially those who are less fit. Unlike cytokine therapies, some of the targeted agents (Sutent and Torisel) have been shown to extend survival with acceptable toxicity, regardless of age. A recent study of Nexavar showed a somewhat greater benefit in elderly patients than in the younger patients. Advanced age did not seem to affect side effects like fatigue, anemia, or skin problems. On the other hand, studies of Torisel and Avastin showed that the severity of side effects increased slightly with age.

There is little information available about the risks and benefits of Avastin in older patients with kidney cancer, but there does appear to be an increased risk of blood clots and other vascular problems with Avastin, especially in those with hypertension or cardiovascular problems. Gastrointestinal side effects (including bowel obstruction and perforation) can be especially troublesome in older patients who are predisposed to constipation.

Though the side effects of cancer treatment are never less burdensome in the elderly, they can be managed by oncologists, especially geriatric oncologists, who work in teams with others who specialize in the care of the elderly. With appropriate care, healthy older patients do just as well with chemotherapy as younger patients. Advances in supportive care (antinausea medicines and blood cell growth factors) have significantly decreased the side effects of systemic therapy and improved safety and the quality of life of individuals with kidney cancer. Nonetheless, there is risk, especially if the patient is frail. The presence of severe comorbidities, age-related frailty, or underlying severe psychosocial problems may be obstacles for highly intensive treatment plans. Such patients may benefit from less-complicated or potentially less-toxic treatment plans.

COMMON TREATMENT COMPLICATIONS IN THE ELDERLY

Anemia (low red blood cell count) is common in the elderly, especially the frail elderly. It decreases the effectiveness of chemotherapy and often causes fatigue, falls, cognitive decline (for example, dementia, disorientation, or confusion), and heart problems. Therefore, it is essential that anemia be recognized and corrected with red blood cell transfusions or the appropriate use of erythropoiesis-stimulating agents like Procrit, Epogen, or Aranesp.

Myelosuppression (decrease in blood counts including low white blood cell count) is also common in older patients getting systemic therapy or radiation therapy. Older patients with myelosuppression develop life-threatening infections more often than younger patients, and they may need to be treated in the hospital for many days. The liberal use of granulopoietic growth factors (G-CSF, Neupogen, Neulasta) decreases the risk of infection.

Mucositis (mouth sores) and **diarrhea** can cause severe **dehydration** in older patients who often are already dehydrated due to an inadequate fluid intake and diuretics ("water pills" for high blood pressure or heart failure). Careful monitoring and the liberal use of antidiarrheal agents (Imodium) and oral and intravenous fluids are essential components of the management of older cancer patients, especially those receiving Nexavar or Sutent.

Kidney function declines as we age. Some of the medicines that older patients take to treat both their cancer (for example, Reclast/Zometa, NSAIDs) and noncancer–related problems might make this worse. The dehydration that often accompanies cancer and its treatment can put additional stress on the kidneys. Obviously, this is even more of a problem in those who have had a nephrectomy. Fortunately, it is often possible to minimize these effects by carefully selecting and dosing appropriate drugs, managing "polypharmacy," and preventing dehydration.

Neurotoxicity and **cognitive effects ("chemo brain")** can be profoundly debilitating in patients who are already cognitively impaired (demented, disoriented, confused, etc.). Elderly patients with a history of falling, hearing loss, or peripheral neuropathy (nerve damage from, for example, diabetes) have decreased energy and are highly vulnerable to neurotoxic chemotherapy like Intron A/Roferon A and Proleukin. Many of the medicines used to control nausea (antiemetics) or decrease the side effects of certain chemotherapeutic agents are also potential neurotoxins. These include dexamethasone (psychosis and agitation), ranitidine (agitation), Benadryl, and some of the antiemetics (sedation).

Fatigue is a near universal complaint of older cancer patients. It is particularly a problem for those who are socially isolated or depend upon others to help them with activities of daily living. It is not necessarily related to **depression**, but can be. Depression is quite common in the elderly. In contrast to younger patients who often respond to a cancer diagnosis with anxiety, depression is the more common disorder in older cancer patients. Intron A/Roferon A can also cause it. With proper support and medical attention, many of these patients can safely receive anticancer treatment.

Heart problems increase with age, and it is no surprise that older cancers patients have an increased risk of cardiac complications from many anticancer agents. Hypertension (high blood pressure) is often a problem when targeted therapy is given, and congestive heart failure and edema (leg swelling or "water on the lungs") are common side effects of cytokine therapy.

Skin problems (including rash, peeling skin, and itching) can occur with any systemic treatment, but these problems are more common with the targeted therapies. The early use of topical moisturizing agents can minimize skin toxicity.

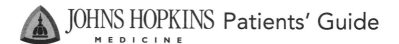

CHAPTER 11

JOHNS HOPKINS Patients' Guide
MEDICINE

TRUSTED RESOURCES—FINDING ADDITIONAL INFORMATION ABOUT KIDNEY CANCER AND ITS TREATMENT

National Cancer Institute

http://www.cancer.gov/cancerinfo

This website offers educational information for patients and family members seeking information about kidney cancer. This links to the same website as the Cancer Information Service.

American Cancer Society

1-800-ACS-2345

http://www.cancer.org

The ACS website has educational information about kidney cancer.

Cancer Information Service of the National Cancer Institute

1-800-4-CANCER

http://www.cancer.gov/cancertopics/types/kidney

This website provides information about all types of cancer including excellent information about kidney cancer, what it is, how it is treated, and where various treatment options are provided. You can request free information by calling the toll-free number.

Kidney Cancer Association

1-800-850-9132

http://www.kidneycancer.org

Email: office@kidneycancer.org

This organization provides information about kidney cancer in the three primary areas of focus: education, research, and advocacy. The website has a wealth of kidney cancer specific information and resources for patients and families.

Urology Health

http://urologyhealth.org/search

This organization has information about kidney cancer and a printable booklet. It can also help you find an urologist through a link to the American Urological Association Foundation.

Oncology Nursing Society

http://www.cancersymptoms.org

This website provides helpful information about managing the side effects of cancer and its treatments.

National Hospice and Palliative Care Organization

http://www.nhpco.org

This organization provides specific information about end-of-life care to maintain quality of life and reduce suffering.

WHERE CAN I GET HELP WITH FINANCIAL OR LEGAL CONCERNS?

Accompanying any serious illness are questions and concerns related to expenses incurred as a result of treatment, health insurance questions that can be overwhelming to try to understand or resolve alone, and sometimes even legal questions related to employment or financial matters. The following is a list of national resources to aid you in addressing these types of concerns.

Cancer Care, Inc.

1-212-302-2400

1-800-813-HOPE

http://www.cancercare.org

Email: info@cancercare.org

Cancer Care is a national nonprofit organization that provides free, professional assistance to people with any type of cancer and to their families. This organization offers education, one-on-one counseling, financial assistance for non-medical expenses, and referrals to community services.

National Coalition for Cancer Survivorship

   1-301-650-8868

   1-877-NCSS-YES

   http://www.canceradvoocy.org

This network of independent groups and individuals provides information and resources about cancer support, advocacy, and quality-of-life issues as well as helps cancer patients deal with insurance or job discrimination and other related legal matters.

Patient Advocate Foundation

   1-757-873-6668

   1-800-532-5274

   http://www.patientadvocate.org

   Email: patient@pinn.net

This organization provides general educational information about managed care/insurance issues and legal counseling on debt intervention, job discrimination issues, and insurance denials of coverage.

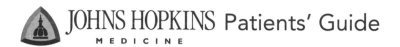 **JOHNS HOPKINS** Patients' Guide
MEDICINE

INFORMATION ABOUT JOHNS HOPKINS

About the James Buchanan Brady Urological Institute
http://urology.jhu.edu

Endowed by James Buchanan Brady, the Brady Buchanan Urological Institute is recognized worldwide as a leader in the discovery and management of urologic diseases. The Brady Institute is consistently ranked by *U.S. News & World Report* as the #1 urology department in the country and offers comprehensive care for patients with kidney cancer.

About the Sidney Kimmel Comprehensive Cancer Center at Johns Hopkins

http://www.hopkinskimmelcancercenter.org

Since its inception in 1973, the Sidney Kimmel Comprehensive Cancer Center at Johns Hopkins has been dedicated to better understanding human cancers and finding more effective treatments. One of only forty cancer centers in the country designated by the National Cancer Institute (http://www.cancer.gov) as a Comprehensive Cancer Center, the Johns Hopkins Kimmel Cancer Center has active programs in clinical research, laboratory research, education, community outreach, and prevention and control and is the only Comprehensive Cancer Center in the state of Maryland.

About Johns Hopkins Medicine

http://hopkinsmedicine.org

Johns Hopkins Medicine unites physicians and scientists of the Johns Hopkins University School of Medicine with the organizations, health professionals, and facilities of the Johns Hopkins Health System. Its mission is to improve the health of the community and the world by setting the standard of excellence in medical education, research, and clinical care. Diverse and inclusive, Johns Hopkins Medicine has provided international leadership in the education of physicians and medical scientists in biomedical research and in the application of medical knowledge to sustain health since The Johns Hopkins Hospital opened in 1889.

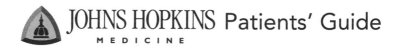

FURTHER READING

100 Questions & Answers About Kidney Cancer by Steven C. Campbell, MD, PhD; Brian I. Rini, MD; Robert G. Uzzo, MD, FACS; Brian R. Lane, MD, PhD; and Stephanie Chisolm, PhD. Jones and Bartlett Publishers, 2009.

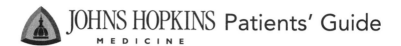

JOHNS HOPKINS Patients' Guide

MEDICINE

GLOSSARY

Adjuvant therapy: Treatment given after the primary treatment to increase the chances of a cure, and treatment to prevent the cancer from recurring.

Advance directives: Legal documents that allow people to express their decisions regarding what they do and don't want to have done during their last weeks or months in case they become unable to communicate effectively.

Alopecia: Hair loss that can be complete or just a thinning of scalp hair.

Alternative therapy: Medicines used in lieu of standard medical therapies.

Anemia: Low level of red blood cells that contain hemoglobin (an iron protein) that provides oxygen to all parts of the body.

Antiemetics: Antinausea medications.

Arterial embolization: The placement of a special sponge-like material into an artery that is supplying blood to the kidney involved with the cancer.

Biopsy: A procedure in which cells are collected for microscopic examination.

Bisphosphonate: Medicine that strengthens bones.

Bone scan: A type of X-ray that can identify signs of metastasis in the bones.

Cancer: The presence of malignant cells.

Cancer survivor: A person who survives cancer from the time of diagnosis until present, including people who are suffering from terminal forms of the disease. This also includes family members, friends, and caregivers of those who have been diagnosed.

Carcinomas: Cancers that form in the surface cells of different tissues.

Cells: Basic elements of tissues; the appearance and composition of individual cells are unique to the tissue they compose.

Chemotherapy: The use of chemical agents (drugs) to systemically treat cancer.

Chronic pain: Pain that is present for extended periods of time, though not always at the same level of intensity.

Clear-cell carcinoma: A type of kidney cancer that comprises 70 percent of all kidney cancers.

Clinical trial: A study of a drug or treatment with a large group of people testing the treatment.

Cognitive dysfunction: A difficulty with concentration, memory, or arithmetic that can be association with systemic treatment and stress; "chemo brain."

Complementary therapy: Medicines used in conjunction with standard therapies.

Cryoablation or cryosurgery: Involves freezing the tumor to kill the cancer cells using liquid nitrogen or carbon dioxide.

Cytotoxic: The ability to kill fast-growing cells, both cancerous and noncancerous, by preventing them from dividing.

Durable power of attorney: A document that specifies a family member to have legal authority to make all decisions, personal and financial, for you (usually based on prior discussions of wishes) in case you become incapacitated.

Fine-needle aspiration biopsy: A procedure in which a very thin needle is used to collect fluid or cells directly from the mass for evaluation.

Genetic mutation: A gene with a mistake or alteration.

Guided imagery: A mind-body technique in which the patient visualizes and meditates on images that encourage a positive immune response.

Hand-foot syndrome: A condition in which the skin on the palms of the hands and soles of the feet becomes red and inflamed; blistering and peeling can occur.

Heathcare proxy: A document that permits a designated person to make decisions regarding your medical treatment when you are unable to do so.

Hereditary kidney cancer: Kidney cancer that is linked to genetic changes.

Histologic tumor grade: Describes how slow or fast the cancer is growing; how aggressive the cancer is and may progress from stage to stage.

Hospice: Approaches and support to help with end-of-life care, including personal care, symptom control, and quality of life. End-of-life care may occur at home or in an inpatient hospice setting; hospice providers can also help with bereavement issues for the patient and family.

Hypercalcemia: An accelerated loss of calcium in the bones, leading to elevated levels of the mineral in the bloodstream with symptoms such as nausea and confusion.

Immunotherapy: Treatment given to stimulate the body's immune system in order to fight disease.

Incidence: The number of times a disease occurs within a population of people.

Informed consent: A process by which patients participating in a specific treatment or clinical study are provided with all the available information regarding the experimental treatment prior to consenting to receive that treatment.

Initial therapy: Treatment given as the first approach. In kidney cancer, it is usually surgery.

Intraoperative radiation: A dose of radiation is given directly to the tumor site immediately after the surgery to remove the tumor.

Invasive cancer: Cancer that grows and invades into areas surrounding the initial site where the cancer started.

Laparoscopic nephrectomy: Minimally invasive surgical technique that involves inserting an instrument (laparoscope) into the abdominal cavity via small incisions to remove part or all of the kidney.

Laparoscopy: Minimally invasive surgical technique that is performed by inserting an instrument (laparoscope) into the abdomen via small incisions to remove surgical proceudure.

Living will: A document that outlines what care you want in the event you are no longer able to let your wishes be known due to coma or heavy sedation.

Lymph: Fluid carried through the body by the lymphatic system, composed primarily of white blood cells and diluted plasma.

Lymph nodes: Tissues in the lymphatic system that filter lymph fluid and help the immune system fight disease.

Lymphatic system: A collection of vessels with the principal functions of transporting digested fat from the intestine to the bloodstream, removing and destroying toxins from tissues, and resisting the spread of disease throughout the body.

Malignant: Cancerous; growing rapidly and out of control.

Medical oncologist: *See* oncologist.

Metastasis, metastasize: The spread of cancer to other organ sites.

Mortality: The statistical calculation of death rates dues to a specific disease within a population.

Mucositis: Inflammation and sores in the mouth and throat usually from systemic therapy.

Mutated: Altered.

Neoadjuvant therapy: Adjuvant therapy that is started before the primary treatment.

Nephrectomy: Surgical removal of the entire kidney.

Neutropenia: A condition of an abnormally low number of a particular type of white blood cell called a neutrophil. White blood cells (leukocytes) are the cells in the blood that play important roles in fighting off infection.

Noninvasive cancer: Cancer confined to its tissue point of origin and not found in surrounding tissue.

Nonsteroidal anti-inflammatory drugs (NSAIDs): A class of pain medications, often sold over the counter, that includes ibuprofen and similar common pain killers.

Oncologist: A cancer specialist who helps determine treatment choices, primarily with drugs or medications.

Open procedures: Surgical procedures where an incision is made to visualize the organs and tissue to be removed.

Open radical nephrectomy: A surgical procedure performed through a large incision that removes the kidney and surrounding tissue.

Opioids: Medicines derived from morphine and similar chemicals (narcotics).

Palliative care: Care to relieve the symptoms of cancer and to keep the best quality of life for as long as possible when a cure is no longer the goal.

Papillary carcinoma: A type of kidney cancer that is the second most common, making up 10–15 percent of kidney cancers.

Pathologist: A specialist trained to distinguish normal from abnormal cells.

Peripheral neuropathy: Damage to the peripheral nerves that can result in numbness, loss of sensation, pain, and mobility problems, usually in the fingers and toes initially but can progress up the extremity.

Persistent pain: Pain that is present for extended periods of time, though not always at the same level intensity.

Partial laparoscopic nephrectomy: Removal of a portion of the kidney or only the area involved with the cancer via laparoscopy (inserting an instrument [laparoscope] into the abdominal cavity via small incisions).

Partial nephrectomy: Surgical removal of a portion of the kidney; removal of the only the area involved with the cancer.

Phases: A series of steps followed in clinical trials to test and develop a new drug or combination of drugs.

> phase I aims to define the tolerated dose, safety, and toxicity of a new drug or new combination of drugs

> phase II aims to define how effective a new drug or combination is in treating a specific disease and to further define safety and toxicity

> phase III aims to define how effective a new drug or combination is when compared with the current standard treatment for a specific disease

Placebos: Treatment or pills that have no treatment benefit given in some clinical trials to determine the effect of a new treatment; often referred to as "sugar pills."

Platelets: Components of blood that assist in clotting and wound healing.

Primary care doctor: Family physician or internist who gives regular medical check-ups and treatment of noncancer-related illness.

Primary prevention: Any treatment method or lifestyle change that directly prevents cancer cells from forming, growing, or multiplying.

Primary treatment/therapy: The initial treatment for kidney cancer; usually involves surgery.

Prognosis: An estimation of the likely outcome of an illness based upon the patient's current status and the available treatments.

Protocol: The treatment plan that can be research and provides information about how, when, and to whom a drug or treatment is given.

Radiation oncologist: A cancer specialist who determines the amount of radiotherapy required.

Radiation physicist: A person who makes sure that the equipment is working properly and that the machines deliver the correct dose of radiation.

Radiation therapist: A person who positions the patients for radiation treatments and runs the equipment that delivers the radiation.

Radiation therapy: Use of high-energy X-rays to kill cancer cells and shrink tumors.

Radical laparoscopic nephrectomy: Removal of the entire kidney and surrounding tissue; may include the removal of the adrenal gland, lymph nodes close to the kidney, and portion of the renal vein or vena cava via laparoscopy (inserting an instrument [laparoscope] into the abdominal cavity via small incisions).

Radical nephrectomy: Removal of the entire kidney and surrounding tissue; may include the removal of the adrenal gland, lymph nodes close to the kidney, and portion of the renal vein or vena cava.

Radiofrequency ablation: Use of high-frequency alternating current to create frictional heat within the tumor to "burn" the tumor cells to death without the need to actually surgically remove them.

Radiologist: A physician specializing in the diagnosis of disease using radiology tests such as X-ray, scans, and the like.

Radiosurgery ablation: Uses robotic devices and imaging software to target specific areas with high-energy beams of radiation.

Recurrent cancer: The disease has come back in spite of the initial treatment.

Red blood cells: Cells in the blood with the primary function of carrying oxygen to tissues.

Risk factors: Any factors that contribute to an increased possibility of getting cancer.

Robotic-assisted surgery: Minimally invasive surgical procedure in which the surgeon sits at a remote console and uses robotic arms and a laparoscope-type instrument to guide the procedure through a small incision.

Sarcomas: Cancers that form in connective tissues.

Secondary prevention: Treatments or lifestyle changes that limit a person's exposure to cancer risk factors, but don't directly prevent the formation of cancer.

Sexual dysfunction: Difficulty with sexual function that can encompass impotence (lack of erection), loss of lubrication, painful intercourse, or a loss of interest in sex.

Stage: A numerical determination to define how far the cancer has progressed.

Stomatitis: Inflammation and sores of the mouth and throat usually from systemic therapy.

Surgical biopsy: Removes a portion of the tissue for further evaluation and diagnosis.

Surgical oncologist: A specialist trained in the surgical removal of cancerous tumors.

Systemic treatment: A treatment that travels to all parts of the body, such as oral or intravenous treatment.

Targeted therapy: Treatment that targets specific molecules or growth pathways involved in tumor growth.

Thrush: Fungal or yeast infection of the mucosa in the mouth.

Tumor: A mass or lump of tissue that is abnormal.

Ultrasonography: A procedure that uses sound waves to determine whether an abnormality exists.

Unilateral: One side.

Urologist: A surgeon who specializes in treating diseases of the genitourinary tract, including cancer of the kidneys, prostate, bladder, and testes.

von Hippel-Lindau (VHL): One type of hereditary kidney cancer that makes up 75 percent of hereditary kidney cancer.

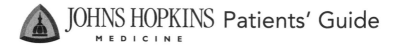

JOHNS HOPKINS Patients' Guide
MEDICINE

INDEX

Adjuvant treatment, 37–38
Adrenal gland, 29
Adrucil (5-fluorouracil), 35, 101
Afinitor (everolimus), 35, 46, 48, 53, 85, 101
Age. *See* older adults
Alcohol, 79
Alopecia, 57–59, 69
American Cancer Society, 81, 107
American College of Surgeons, 3
Americans with Disabilities Act, 64
Anemia, 3, 46–47, 103
Antiemetics, 51, 104
Anzemet (dolasetron), 53
Appetite or taste changes, 54
Appointments navigator, 24
Aranesp (darbepoetin), 46, 103
Arterial embolization, 32, 101
Ativan (lorazepam), 53

Avastin (bevacizumab), 35, 37, 46, 48, 49, 102

Back pain, 3
Benadryl (diphenhydramine), 55, 105
Biopsies, 5, 6–7, 11, 17, 18, 21, 23
Bisphophonates, 86
Blood cell counts, 46, 49, 103
Blood clots, 102
Blood in urine, 2–3, 35, 94
Blood pressure, 3, 48–49
Blood tests, 23
Body image, 58
Bone scan, 23
Boniva (ibandronate), 53
Brain cancer, 84–85, 86
Brain scan, 23

Calcium levels, 3
Cancer Care, Inc., 109

Carcinogens, 94
Cardiac risk, 48, 105
Case managers, 24
CAT (computed axial tomography) scans, 5, 6, 19–20, 23, 84, 95, 96
Chemo brain, 50–51, 104
Chemotherapy, 16, 17, 27, 35, 38, 46, 53, 57, 68, 69, 101, 102, 103, 104
Children, 13, 22, 49–50, 61, 62–63, 68, 70–71, 72, 100
Chromophobe renal-cell carcinomas, 8
Cialis (tadalafil), 60
Clear-cell carcinomas, 2, 8
Clinical staging, 11
Clinical trials, 39–43, 86
Cognitive dysfunction, 50–51, 103, 104
Collecting duct renal-cell carcinomas, 8
Communication
  asking for help, 65
  with boss and coworkers, 64–65
  with parents and siblings, 63–64
  specialists in, 62
  with teens, 63
  using email, 65
  with young children, 62
Comorbidity, 93, 98, 100, 103
Compazine (prochloroperazine), 53
Complete blood count (CBC), 23
Comprehensive metabolic panel, 23
Congestive heart failure, 48, 105
Constipation, 57, 101, 102
Coping, 67–73. *See also* communication

Cortisone cream, 55
Counseling, 76–77
Cryoablation, 31–32, 86, 101
Cytokine therapy, 102, 105

Deep breathing techniques, 79
Dehydration, 52, 104
Dementia, 97, 99, 103
Dental issues, 72–73
Depression, 57, 97, 105
Dexamethasone, 104
Diagnosis, 1–3, 94–95
Diarrhea, 54–55, 71–72, 99, 104

Edema, 105
EKG (echocardiogram), 48
Elavil (amitriptyline), 57
Employment issues, 64–65, 70–71
End of life issues, 87–92
Epogen (epoetin), 46, 103
Erectile dysfunction, 60
Estate planning, 99
Exercise, 78

Family
  communication with, 62–64
  presence at first visit, 20
  stress and, 26, 65, 68
  and treatment for older adults, 97, 99
Family Medical Leave Act (FMLA), 70–71
Fatigue, 46, 47–48, 71–72, 101, 104, 105
Fear of recurrence, 76
Fever, 3, 49, 50
FH (fumarate hydratase) gene, 13
Financial issues, 25–26, 65, 68, 109. *See also* insurance
Fine-needle aspirates, 5
First appointment, 18–23

Flu shots, 73
Fosamax (alendronate), 53
Friends, 59, 65, 97, 99
Fuhrman system, 12

Gemzar (gemcitabine), 35, 101
Genetics, 12–14
Genetics counseling, 3, 13–14
Geriatric oncology programs, 100
Grading, 12
Granulopoietic growth factors (G-GSF), 104

Hair loss, 57–59, 69
Health insurance, 4, 20, 25–26, 43, 58, 109–110
Heart problems, 48, 105
Hemoglobin, 46
Heredity, 12, 13
High blood pressure, 3, 21, 48–49, 98, 104, 105
Hospice/palliative care, 91–92, 97, 101, 109

Image Recovery, 58
Imaging studies, 19–20. *See also* CAT (computed axial tomography) scans; MRI (magnetic resonance imaging); ultrasonography; X-rays
Immunotherapy, 29–30, 35
Imodium (lopcramide), 54, 104
Infection, 49–50, 72–73, 103–104
Initial consultation, 18–23
Initial workup, 23–24
Insurance, 4, 20, 25–26, 43, 58, 109–110
Interferon, or IFN (Intron A, Roferon A), 29–30, 35, 36, 37, 102, 104, 105

Interleukin 2, or IL2 (Proleukin), 29–30, 35, 36, 49, 53, 85, 102, 104

Journaling, 80

Kidney Cancer Association, 4–5, 108
Kytril (granisetron), 53

Laparoscopic surgery, 28, 30–31, 101
LDH test, 23
Legal issues, 99, 109
Leiomyomas, 13
Levitra (vardenafil), 60
Life expectancy, 95–96
Lifestyle changes, 77–79
Lomotil (diphenoxylate and atropine), 55
Look Good, Feel Good program, 58
Lymph nodes, 9, 10, 11–12, 17, 29, 95
Lyrica (pregabalin), 57

Medical history, 21
Medical oncologist, 3, 16
Medical records, 6–7
Meditation, 79
Medullary renal-cell carcinomas (RCC), 8
Metastatic disease, 2, 87–92
MET gene, 13
Mouth sores, 53–54, 104
MRI (magnetic resonance imaging), 6–7, 20, 23, 34
Mucositis, 53–54, 104
MUGA scan, 48
Myelosuppression, 46, 49, 103–104

National Cancer Institute, 3, 107, 108

National Coalition for Cancer Survivorship, 110

National Hospice and Palliative Care Organization, 109

Nausea and vomiting, 51–53, 71

Neoadjuvant treatment, 37, 42

Nephrectomy, 5–6, 28–31, 83, 101, 104

Neulasta, 104

Neupogen, 104

Neurological problems, 56–57

Neurontin (gabapentin), 57

Neurotoxicity, 104–105

Neutropenia, 49

Nexavar (sorafenib), 35, 36, 37, 46, 48, 54, 55, 58, 85, 101, 102, 104

NSAIDS, 104

Nurses, 17

Nutrition, 77–78

Older adults
  clinical trials, 93
  comorbidity, 93, 98, 100, 103
  decision making, 94–99
  increased risk for cancer, 94
  polypharmacy, 93, 98, 104
  prejudice, 93–94
  treatment complications, 103–105
  treatment options, 97–98, 100–103
  treatment team, 99

Oncocytoma renal-cell carcinomas (RCC), 8

Oncology Nursing Society, 48, 108

Open radical nephrectomy, 29

Opioid (narcotic) pain relievers, 101

Pain
  in the bone, 23
  infection and, 49
  of mouth sores, 53
  peripheral neuropathy and, 56
  quality of life and, 89
  radiation and, 16–17, 39, 101
  recurrence and, 84
  of skin rashes, 55
  surgical, 31, 32, 33, 77
  as a symptom, 3

Palliative care, 91–92, 96, 97, 101, 109

Papillary carcinomas, 2, 8, 13

Partial laparoscopic nephrectomy, 30–31, 101

Partial nephrectomy, 28–29

Pathological staging, 11–12

Pathologists, 17, 29, 38

Pathology, 7–8

Patient Advocate Foundation, 110

Patient navigators, 24

Peripheral neuropathy, 56–57, 77, 104–105

Polypharmacy, 93, 98, 104

Post-treatment issues. See survivorship

Preauthorizations, 20

Procrit (epoetin), 46, 103

Psychosocial support staff, 3

Quality-of-life issues
  clinical trials that address, 39, 41, 42
  fatigue, 46, 47–48, 71–72, 101, 104, 105
  hospice/palliative care, 91–92
  metastatic disease, 87, 89
  for older patients, 97, 103
  sexual dysfunction, 59–60
  when to end treatment, 90

Questions
  about clinical trials, 42–43
  to ask urologist, 4
  for initial consultation, 21–23

Radiation oncologists, 3, 16–17
Radiation therapy
  about, 39
  for older adults, 101
  palliative, 89
  for recurrence, 85–86
  side effects, 47, 51–52, 54, 55–
    56, 58, 72
  treatment schedules, 70
Radical nephrectomy, 28–29
Radiofrequency ablation, 31–32,
    35, 86, 101
Radiologists, 3, 17
Rash Relief, 55
Reclast (zolendronic acid), 53,
    86, 104
Records. See medical records
Recurrence, 76, 83–86, 89, 90
Red blood cells (RBCs), 46
Reglan (metaclopramide), 53
Relaxation therapy, 79
Renal-cell carcinomas (RCC), 8
Risk of recurrence, 83–86

Sarcomatoid renal-cell
    carcinomas (RCC), 8
Secondary smoke, 79
Second opinion, 4, 28
Sexual dysfunction, 59–60
Side effects
  anemia, 3, 46–47, 103
  blood pressure, 3, 48–49
  cognitive dysfunction, 50–51,
    104
  diarrhea, 54–55, 71–72, 104
  fatigue, 46, 47–48, 71–72, 101,
    104, 105

hair loss, 57–59
heart problems, 48, 105
infection, 49–50, 72, 103–104
long-term, 77
loss of appetite or taste
    changes, 54
mouth sores, 53–54, 104
nausea and vomiting, 51–53, 71
in older adults, 98, 101, 102,
    103–105
peripheral neuropathy, 56–57,
    104–105
sexual dysfunction, 59–60
skin rashes and effects, 55–56,
    105
Sidney Kimmel Comprehensive
    Cancer Center, 110
Skin rashes and effects, 55–56,
    105
Smoking, 79
Social workers, 17–18, 26
Specialists, 3, 4, 62, 99
Staging, 8–12, 95
Stomatitis, 53–54
Stress, 51, 62, 65, 68, 78–79,
    104
Surgery
  arterial embolization, 32
  cryoblation, 31–32, 35
  laparoscopic, 30–31
  nephrectomy, 5–6, 28
  for older adults, 100–101
  open approach, 28–30
  preoperative instruction, 69
  radiofrequency ablation, 31–32,
    35, 86
  recovery, 33–35
  recurrence and, 85, 86
  risk, 29
  robotic-assisted, 31
  treatment following, 39–43
  vascular, 29

Survivorship
    counseling, 76–77
    living a healthier lifestyle, 77–79
    managing long-term side effects, 77
    new perspectives on life, 80–81
    setting new goals, 79–80
Sutent (sunitinib), 35, 36, 37, 46, 48, 54, 55, 58, 72, 85, 101, 102, 104
Symptoms
    caused by kidney cancer, 2–3
    of cognitive dysfunction, 50–51
    of heart problems, 48
    of infection, 49–50
Symptoms (*cont.*)
    of neurological problems, 56–57
    in older adults, 94–96
    palliative care and, 91
    recurrence and, 84, 89, 90
    of sexual dysfunction, 59–60
    of skin rashes, 55–56
Systemic treatment
    adjuvant, 37–38
    chemotherapy, 35–36, 46, 53, 69, 102, 103
    in the elderly, 102
    immunotherapy, 29–30, 35
    neoadjuvant, 37
    planning for, 69
    for recurrence, 85
    targeted therapy, 35, 36–37, 85, 101

Targeted therapy, 35, 36–37, 85, 101
Tegretol (carbamazepine), 57

TNM classification, 9–10
Torisel (temsirolimus), 35, 36, 46, 48, 53, 55, 85, 101, 102
Transitional renal-cell carcinomas, 8
Treatment center, 3
Treatment team, 3, 15–18, 24, 100
Tumor grade, 12

Ultrasonography, 5, 20
Unclassified renal-cell carcinomas, 8
Urinalysis, 23
Urologic pathologists, 3
Urologic surgical oncologist, 15–16
Urologists, 3–4
Urology Health, 108

Vaginal dryness, 60
Vascular surgery, 29
Viagra (sildenfil), 60
Volunteering, 81
Vomiting, 51–53, 71
Von Hippel-Lindau disease (VHL), 12–13

Weight loss, 3, 53
White blood cells, 49, 72, 73, 103
Wigs, 58
Wills, 99
Workplace issues, 64–65, 70–71

Xeloda (capecitabine), 35, 101
X-rays, 6–7, 17, 23, 34, 84

Zofran (ondansetron), 53
Zometa (zolendronic acid), 53, 86, 104